Face Transplantation

Juan P. Barret · Veronica Tomasello

Face Transplantation

Principles, Techniques and Artistry

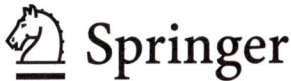

Juan P. Barret, MD, PhD
Department of Plastic Surgery
and Burns
University Hospital Vall d´Hebron
Barcelona
Spain

Veronica Tomasello, MD
Cannizzaro Hospital
Catania
Italy

ISBN 978-3-662-51243-2   ISBN 978-3-662-45444-2   (eBook)
DOI 10.1007/978-3-662-45444-2
Springer Berlin Heidelberg New York Dordrecht London

Printed on acid-free paper

Springer is part of Springer Science+Business Media (www.springer.com)

To my wife Esther and my daughter Júlia, who made all this possible.
Sóu poesia per a la meva vida, amor fins l'infinit. Gràcies per existir

Juan P. Barret, MD, PhD

To Dr. Barret. With all my gratitude for believing in this project.
Non avrei potuto desiderare niente di più e niente di meglio per la mia carriera

Veronica Tomasello, MD

Preface

Reconstructive allotransplantation has emerged as the ultimate restorative technique for treating face deformity, hand amputations and others. In particular, a real revolution in face reconstruction has occurred. The not-so-old dream of restorative surgery, namely the replacement of damaged parts of the body by new, unharmed preformed tissues, has become a reality. The development of techniques aimed towards the transplantation of vascularised composite tissues has provided clinicians with a new, robust tool for the reconstruction of deformities that were, not so long ago, impossible to achieve. The results of face transplantation in humans demonstrate that face transplantation is no longer an abstraction but a clinical reality. It has been implemented in the recent years with increasing interest and great success. The limits of indications are still, though, desperate catastrophic face disfigurement. Similarly to that learnt in many other transplant and plastic surgery disciplines, the development of face transplantation programmes calls for a strong team approach. Building a multidisciplinary team involves joining together all essential and diverse specialists to make a robust protocol and an experienced team that warrants excellency in outcomes. The general objective of our intense efforts in basic, clinical research and implementation in the human clinic is the standardisation and introduction of a new treatment for patients suffering from severe face deformities and destructions caused by burns, trauma, congenital defects and the extirpation of malignant tumours. It introduces technical aspects; immunological, psychological, ethical and legal methodologies; and the necessary surgical proficiency for the performance of face transplantation. With the development of novel, more effective, immunosuppressant regimens, which shall decrease the advent of toxic side effects, the indications for this new technique may widen. In fact, the achievement of such a regimen that minimised side effects and counterbalanced the ethical issues in reconstructive allotransplantation would allow for the transplantation and restoration of any anatomical and functional unit of the human body. Cell therapy, tissue engineering and new synthetic polymers will help in the development of a true restorative surgery in the future, combining the knowledge and expertise of transplantation medicine specialists with the advent and development of biological and synthetic tissue engineering.

Barcelona, Spain   Juan P. Barret, MD, PhD
Catania, Italy   Veronica Tomasello, MD

Contents

Abbreviations

ALT	Alanine aminotransferase
APC	Antigen-presenting cell
ASPS	American Society of Plastic Surgery
AST	Aspartate aminotransferase
atg	Antithymocyte globulin
ATGAM	Equine antilymphocyte globulin
AZA	Azathioprine
BUN	Blood urea nitrogen
CCNE	Comité Consultatif National d'Ethique
CMV	Cytomegalovirus
CNIS	Calcineurin inhibitors
CsA	Cyclosporine
CT	Computed tomography
CTA	Composite tissue allotransplantation
VCA	Vascularised composite tissue allotransplantation
DIEAP	Deep inferior epigastric artery perforator
DSA	Donor-specific antibody
EBV	Epstein-Barr virus
GCS	Glasgow Coma Score
GGT	Gamma glutamyl transpeptidase
GVHD	Graft-versus-host disease
H&E	Hematoxylin and eosin
HDL	High-density lipoprotein
HIV	Human immunodeficiency virus
HLA	Human leukocyte antigen
HTLV	Human T-lymphotrophic virus
HVGR	Host-versus-graft reaction
ICAM	Intercellular adhesion molecule
ICU	Intensive care unit
IFN	Interferon
Ig	Immunoglobulin
IL	Interleukin
IRB	Institutional Review Board
ITU	Intensive therapy unit
IV	Intravenous
LDL	Low-density lipoprotein
MCC	Meningococcal C polysaccharide

MHC	Major histocompatibility complex
MICA	MHC class I chain gene A
MINI	Mini-International Neuropsychiatric Interview
MMF	Mycophenolate mofetil
MMSE	Mini Mental State Exam
MPA	Mycophenolic acid
MRSA	Methicillin-resistant *Staphylococcus aureus*
NG	Nasogastric
NK	Natural killer
PAS	Periodic acid–Schiff
PCR	Polymerase chain reaction
PEEP	Positive end respiratory pressure
PEG	Percutaneous endoscopic gastrostomy
PMN	Polymorphonuclear neutrophil
PPD	Purified protein derivative
RAD	Everolimus
RAPA	Rapamycin
r-ATG	Antithymocytic globulin from rabbits
REC	Research Ethics Committee
SALT	Skin-associated lymphoid tissues
SOT	Solid organ transplantation
SSOP	Specific-sequencing of oligonucleotide primer
SSP	Sequence-specific primer
TGF	Transforming growth factor
TNF	Tumor necrosis factor
TPTA	Activated partial prothrombin time
VCA	Composite vascularised allograft
VCAM	Vascular adhesion molecule
VLDL	Very low density lipoprotein
WMA	World Medical Association

Introduction and General Background

Abstract

The last years have registered an important activity in the specialty of plastic and reconstructive surgery. In particular, a real revolution in reconstruction has occurred. The not-so-old dream of restorative surgery, namely, the replacement of damaged parts of the body by new unharmed preformed tissues, has become a reality. The development of techniques aimed at transplantation of vascularised composite tissues (VCA, vascularised composite allografts) has provided clinicians with a new robust tool for the reconstruction of deformities that were, not so long ago, impossible to achieve. History, development and classical attempts for VCA are not a new one. More than four decades ago, doctors in Ecuador attempted the transplantation of a hand limb. The transplant failed, but the dream survived. Pioneering laboratory work in experimental animals showed the path to clinicians for the achievement of human VCA. The works of Dr. Siemionow and Dr. Butler are milestones of the development of this discipline. They showed how tissues could survive after transplantation and implemented the basis for the surgical technique in the clinical scenario. More than ever, this is a perfect example of translational research and implementation of bench work to the bedside.

The last years have registered an important activity in the specialty of plastic and reconstructive surgery. In particular, a real revolution in reconstruction has occurred. The not-so-old dream of restorative surgery, namely, the replacement of damaged parts of the body by new unharmed preformed tissues, has become a reality. The development of techniques aimed at transplantation of vascularised composite tissues (VCA, vascularised composite allografts) has provided clinicians with a new robust tool for the reconstruction of deformities that were, not so long ago, impossible to achieve. History, development and classical attempts for VCA are not a new one. More than four decades ago, doctors in Ecuador attempted the transplantation of a hand limb. The transplant failed, but the dream survived. Pioneering laboratory work in experimental animals showed the path to clinicians for the achievement of human VCA. The works of

J.P. Barret, V. Tomasello, *Face Transplantation: Principles, Techniques and Artistry*,
DOI 10.1007/978-3-662-45444-2_1, © Springer-Verlag Berlin Heidelberg 2015

Dr. Siemionow and Dr. Butler are milestones of the development of this discipline. They showed how tissues could survive after transplantation and implemented the basis for the surgical technique in the clinical scenario. More than ever, this is a perfect example of translational research and implementation of bench work to the bedside. Not so long ago, Dr. Pribaz et al. at Harvard and Brigham and Women's Hospital illuminated the plastic surgery community with the revolutionary concepts of flap prelamination and prefabrication. These elaborated techniques, well documented in literature, pursue the goal of fabricating new flaps and parts in the human body ready for autotransplantation. There is no surprise that few years later the same institution is at the forefront of face VCA in the USA. On the other hand, VCA has opened a new era not only in reconstructive surgery but also in transplant surgery. To date, there have been reports of successful transplantations of the knee joint, hand (unilateral and bilateral), arms (unilateral and bilateral), face (partial and total), abdominal wall, larynx, penis, digits and lower limbs. All recipients presented with deformities and/or amputations that were not amenable to be reconstructed by means of classical or traditional techniques. Such deformities affected nonvital parts and/or organs, and all of them had in common the impossibility to restore form, function and cosmesis by means of conventional techniques and reconstructive surgery. The results of face transplantation in humans demonstrate that face transplantation is no longer an abstraction but a clinical reality. It has been implemented in the latest years with increasing interest and great success. The limits of indications are still, though, desperate catastrophic face disfigurement. Today, we are in a position to say that it has been possible to perform face transplantation both in animals and humans in a short period of time.

Similarly to that learnt in many other transplant and plastic surgery disciplines, the development of face transplantation programs calls for a strong team approach, building a multidisciplinary team that involves all necessary and diverse specialists to make a robust protocol and an experienced team that warrants excellency in outcomes. This multidisciplinary team is formed by all transplant disciplines usually involved in transplant medicine (surgeons, immunologists, infectious disease specialists, renal disease specialists) but should include also experienced health professionals more involved in the plastic and reconstructive scenario, namely, rehabilitation specialists, physiotherapists, occupational therapists, psychologists, psychiatrists and social workers. VCA procedures must be organised in tertiary centres with a strong commitment to transplant surgery and medicine. Such institutions have in common the required laboratory, clinical services and research units that are necessary to perform this new clinical discipline.

The general objective of our intense efforts in basic, clinical research and implementation in the human clinic is the standardisation and introduction of a new treatment for patients suffering from severe face deformities and destructions caused by burns, trauma, congenital defects and the extirpation of malignant tumours. It introduces technical aspects, immunological, psychological, ethical and legal methodologies and the necessary surgical proficiency for the performance of face transplantation.

1.1   General Aspects

The face has important functional and aesthetic roles. Phylogenetically related, the face has delicate structures to host the senses and to allow for correct nutrition and communication with the environment. However, as human beings, the face plays a central role in personal identity and in social interaction. It is well represented in different languages with different words to refer to the face as an organ ("cara", "faç", "faccia") or as an identity ("rostro; faz" or "visage", "viso"). We are what we see in others, and we recognise people by the face construction, the expression of emotions and the psychosocial input that the face imprints into each other. The face incorporates other exigent functions that merge together anatomy and emotions, such as the discourse, the communication competence and the emotional expression. The latter is very significant from the social and psychological standpoint, since the communication with other human beings involves face expression in non-verbal communication. Its consequences are the following: the importance of the reconstruction of both anatomy and function is fundamental and accepts no controversy, and this requires the application of meticulous and innovative techniques, although total recovery of functions, social and emotional recovery and global aesthetical reconstruction remain extremely difficult. The main reason for such difficulty to obtain an optimal reconstruction of function, emotion and aesthetics of the "face–visage" is the highly specialised organisation of the face as an organ, which has to be approached with exigent technique to form function and aesthetics.

Burns, ballistic trauma (gunshots), benign tumours and malformations (neurofibromatosis and vascular malformations) and cancer ablation may produce important face deformities. The whole scope of plastic surgery does apply for the reconstruction of these defects. However, when important functional anatomical structures such as muscle sphincters (orbital, oral) are involved, final outcome is normally less than optimal. In order to obtain good cosmetic and functional results that match those of absent or deformed tissues, texture, colour and elasticity of tissues should be as similar as possible to the original tissues. Traditional reconstructive face surgery includes the utilisation of skin grafts (partial or full thickness), local flaps, tissue expansion, free flaps and face prelamination. Other nonsurgical options may include custommade prosthetic reconstruction. When final, long-term results are analysed at follow-up, the overall results are usually that of a mask-type appearance. Even in experienced hands, when sophisticated techniques have been used, the lack of an effective function, especially of active competent muscle movement, prevents patients from regaining a normal appearance and correct face functions. Patients are confronted on a long, never-ending number of surgical procedures that in many situations render limited outcomes. Reasons for such important concerns

and limitations include technical, anatomical and physiological issues.

The human face is a unique structure in nature, both by its anatomical basis and its function. Specific features such as the nose, mouth and eyelids cannot be reconstructed or transplanted from another part of the human body. Reaching a final, long-lasting solution for these deformities, making the deformed face a human spirit anew, experimental and translational researches for the last 20 years have been dedicated to study the technical, biological, immunological and ethical possibilities of vascularised composite tissue allotransplantation in humans.

This is not a new idea in reconstructive surgery. The most common method for the reconstruction of face defects is the transplantation (auto) of tissues from adjacent or distant parts of the same patient (Figs. 1.1 and 1.2). Local/regional flaps or grafts are commonly used. Microsurgery is necessary if distant tissues are autotransplanted from the same patient (Figs. 1.3 and 1.4). In some instances, though, prosthesis, osteointegration and biomaterials are utilised (Fig. 1.5). There is no doubt regarding the best outcome possible: it is obtained when tissues from neighbouring areas of the face are the donor areas for the defect. However, when we face severe deformities, these tissues may be absent or destroyed. This situation forces surgeons to search for other techniques that can render the desired outcome, which is no other than "restitutio ad integrum" of the face aspect, the face function and the quality of life. Classical, traditional (including sophisticated microvascular tissue transfers) reconstructions fill defects and repair deformities. However, in the majority of cases, they do not provide patients with a satisfactory aspect, since they do not repair the feeling of avoidance and isolation. It is not uncommon for patients to follow a long series of surgical interventions (some require more than 100 operations in a time span of 10–20 years), not obtaining, though, the desired outcome: social and functional reintegration.

In general terms, conventional techniques are the common option when skin coverage is the main goal of the surgical treatment. However, in

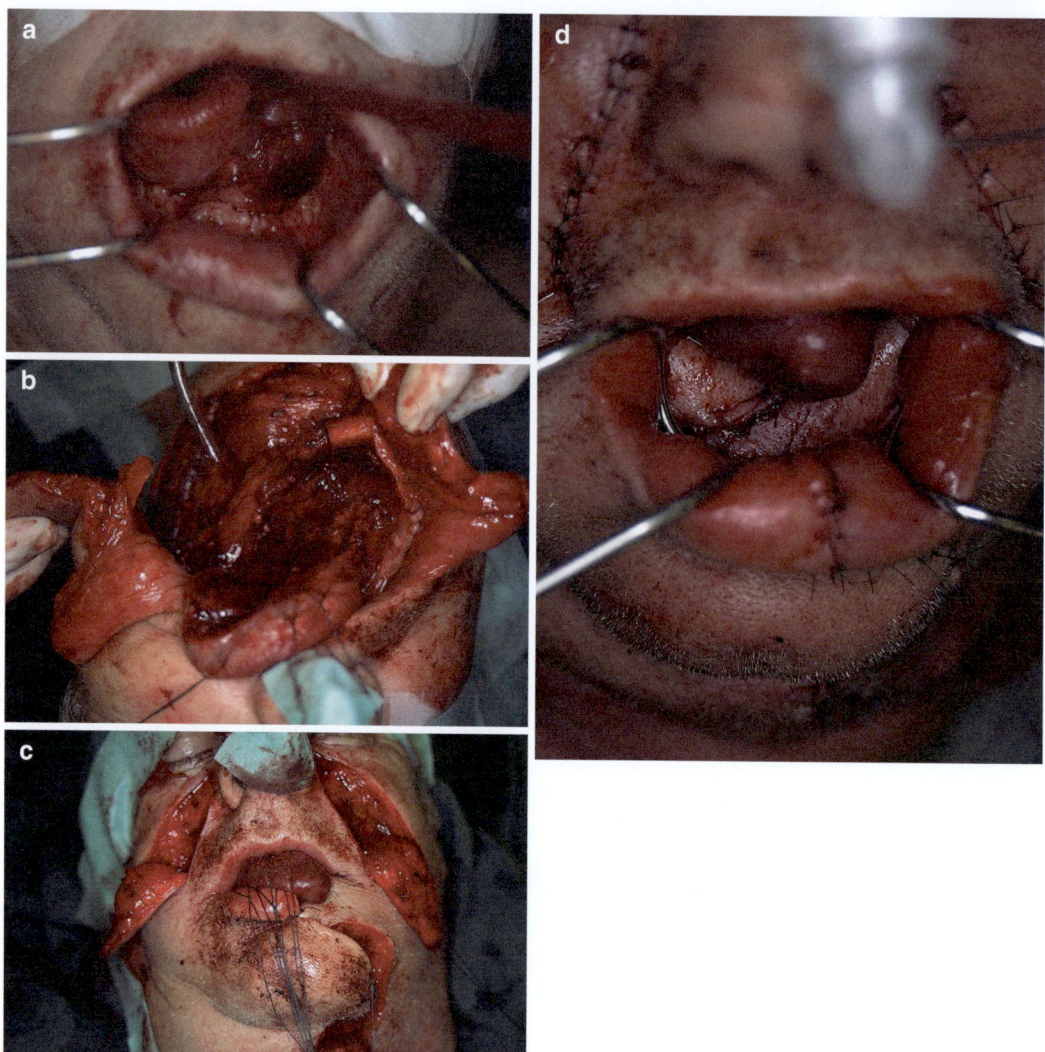

Fig. 1.1 Flap advancement and rotation are workhorses in plastic surgery reconstruction. (**a**) Cancer of the floor of the mouth. (**b**) Defect after resection and mandibular split. (**c**) Nasolabial flaps are elevated to reconstruct the defect. (**d**) Reconstruction with flaps in place

some cases, when extensive damage and severe scars are present and multiple operations with limited outcomes are expected (i.e. burns; Fig. 1.6), face transplantation may be indicated and taken into consideration. It may not improve much the functional outcome of that individual, although it will reintegrate him/her into society and it will avoid multiple conventional operations. Face deformity is a devastating disability

that induces depression, social isolation and risk of suicide. Anger, shyness and avoidance are some of the feelings that face deformity patients feel and receive from society, worsening their recovery after trauma and burns or hindering the adaptation in congenital deformities. Our face is fundamental for physical attraction and is a primary characteristic of our identity. Consequently, a severe deformity, traumatic, innate or acquired,

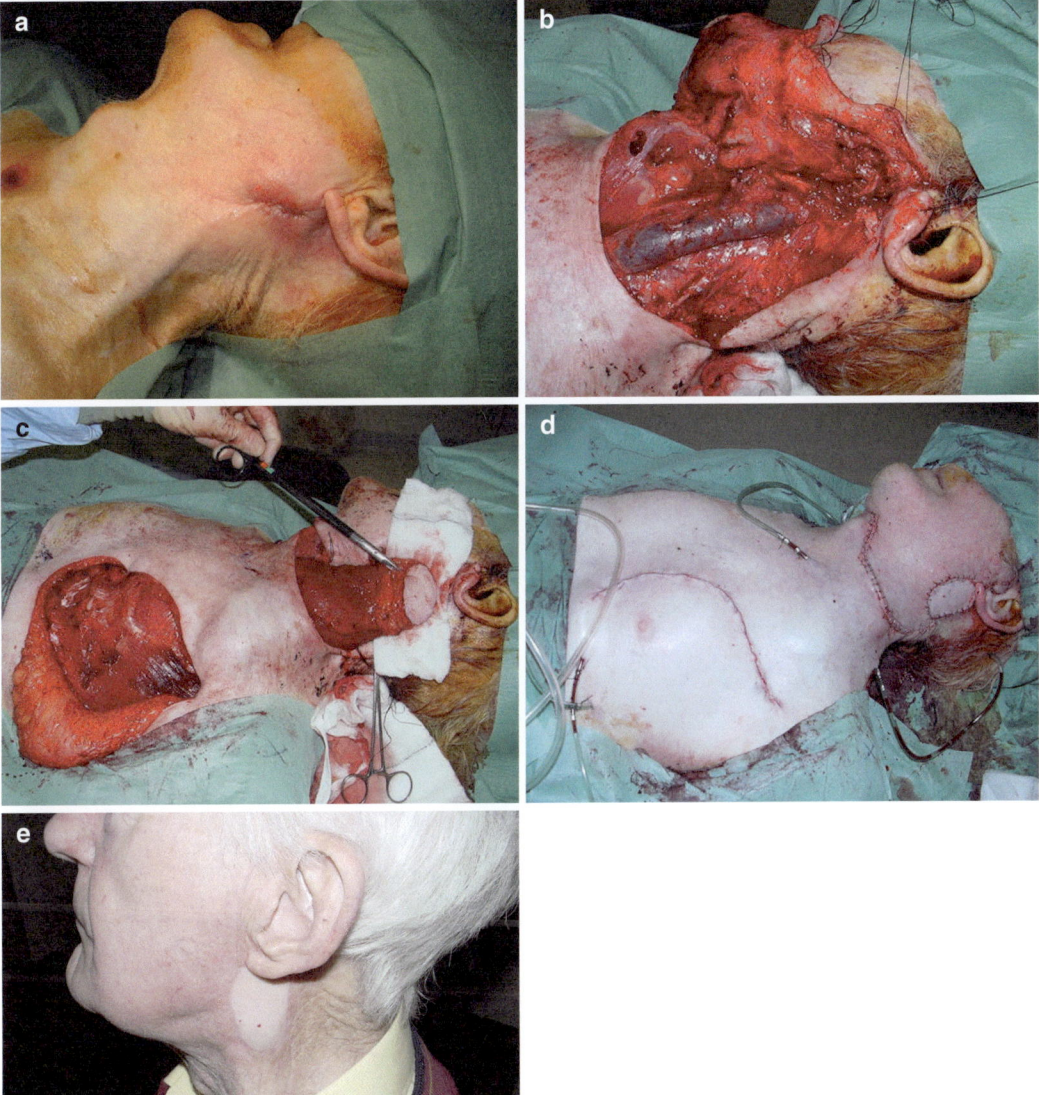

Fig. 1.2 Regional flaps are required when a more complex lesion shall be reconstructed. (**a**) Recurrent parotid tumour involving the cervical skin. (**b**) Defect after resection and modified radical neck dissection. (**c**) Elevation of a pectoralis major myocutaneous flap. (**d**) Result after reconstruction. (**e**) Long-term result

signals that person as "different or diverse". The consequences are social and emotional introversion.

It is estimated that in the USA alone, there are thousands of people that are severely disfigured and live in social isolation and they do not show in public. In general terms, few of them are real candidates for face transplantation. Only those patients that cannot be reconstructed with conventional techniques are candidates for face VCA. On the other hand, it should be stated also that those patients that cannot achieve the same excellent functional outcome offered by face transplantation shall not be offered conven-

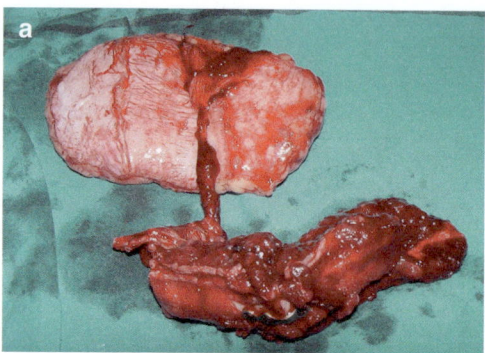
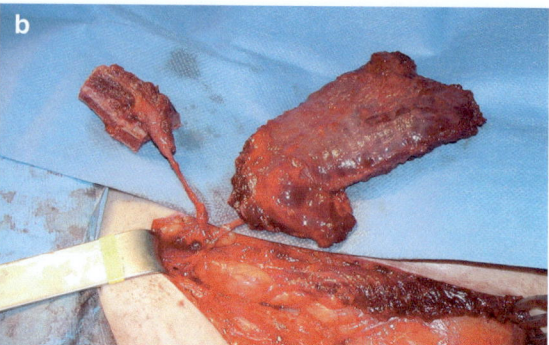

Fig. 1.3 Autotransplantation of flaps/composite tissues is based on reconstructive microsurgery. It joins all important issues in composite tissue allotransplantation with the exception of immunosuppression. (**a**) Free fibula osteocutaneous flap prepared for reconstruction of the mandible and floor of the mouth. Note the preformed fibula with miniplates in place. (**b**) Free deep circumflex iliac artery osteomuscular flap prepared for reconstruction of high-energy traumatism to the forefoot

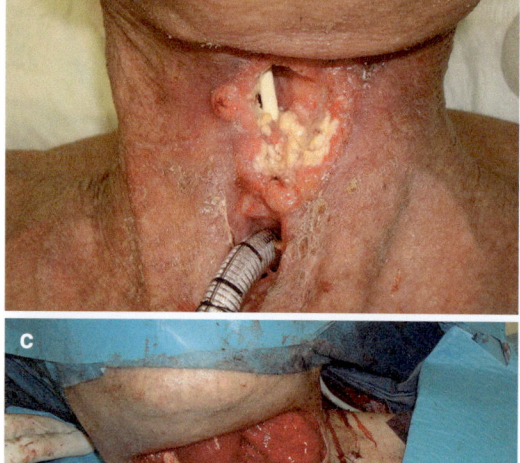
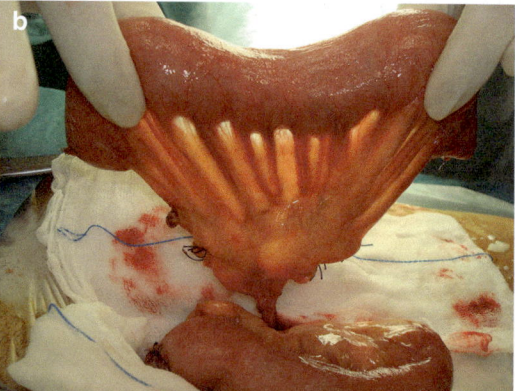
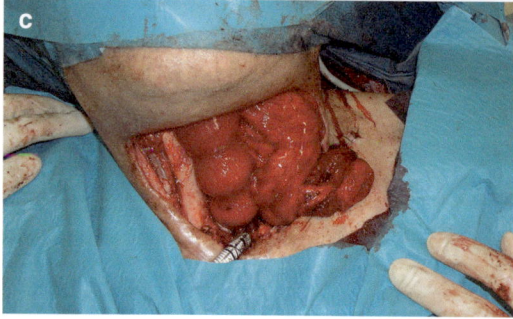

Fig. 1.4 Autotransplantation of a jejunal free flap for the reconstruction of the hypopharynx. (**a**) Recurrent laryngeal tumour after laryngectomy and radiotherapy. (**b**) Preparation of a free jejunal flap. (**c**) Reconstruction of the hypopharynx and oesophagus

tional reconstruction and be evaluated by face transplantation teams. After extirpating all scarred tissues and deformed face units, it is expected that patients recover good functional and aesthetic outcomes in 1–2 years (the time for motor and sensitive nerve recovery). Smiling, laughing, smelling, drinking, eating and speaking shall become again a normal daily living activity, making face transplantation the "gold standard" for these patients.

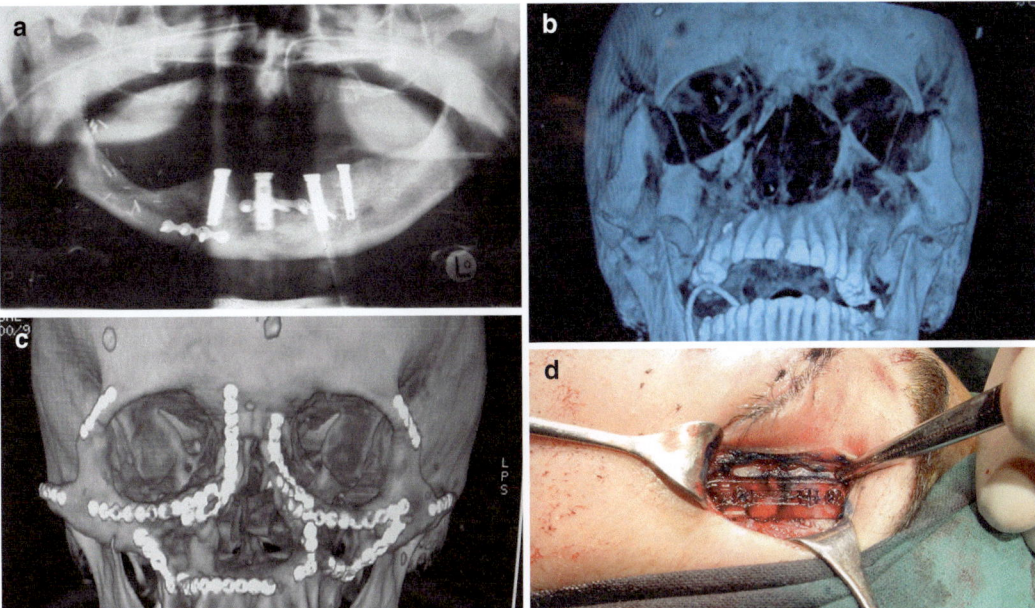

Fig. 1.5 The use of different biomaterials and titanium-based implants aids in craniofacial reconstruction. (**a**) Reconstruccion of a cancer defect of the floor of the mouth a radial forearm free flap and osteointegrated implants. (**b**, **c**) Titanium miniplates are the current foundation for reconstruction of face fractures. (**d**) Resorbable plates are new biomaterials that disappear between 6 months and 1 year

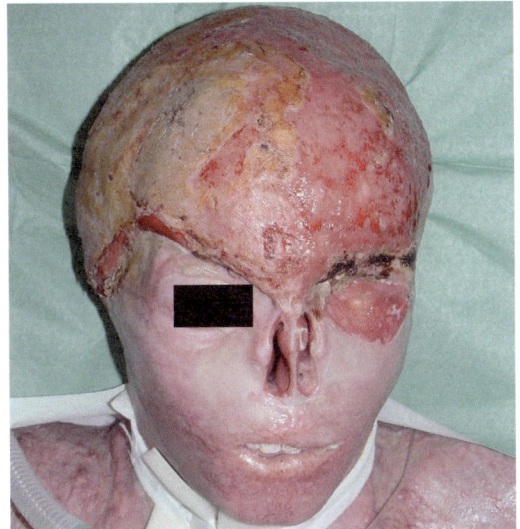

Fig. 1.6 Severe destruction of superficial face structures may indicate face VCA

1.2 Background

The idea of replacing the loss of human anatomical parts (especially limbs) has been depicted by many artists, and it is as old as human history and the history of trauma care. It has been recognised for decades that this objective was far from the human clinic due to immunological and technical barriers. The science behind the immunology of transplantation was initiated with the clinical objective of skin resurfacing and the reconstruction of severely deformed tissues in British pilots and burned navy soldiers injured by U-boat attacks during the Second World War. Physicians such as Tom Gibson and Peter Medawar and other collaborators developed the first experimental studies after tissue immunogenicity, especially skin transplantation and the paradox of

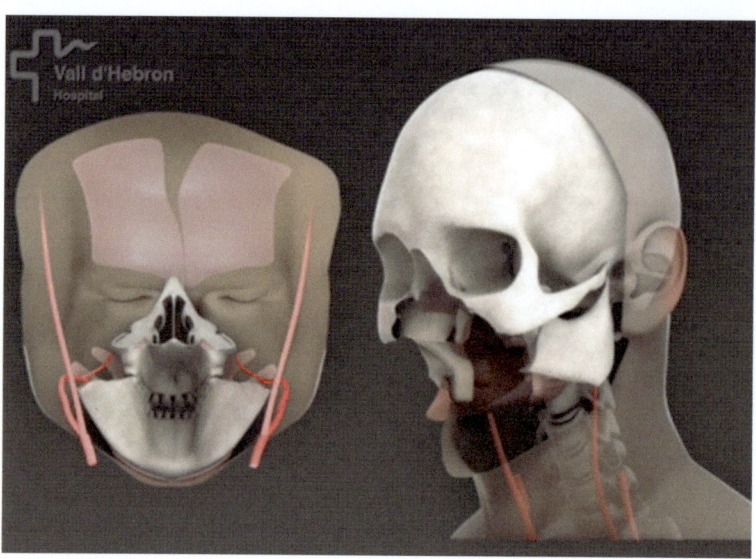

Fig. 1.7 The first full-face transplant performed in March 2010 in Barcelona, Spain

foetal and gestation tolerance. Their work founded the grounds for transplantation and brought a Nobel Prize in 1960. Soon afterwards many other pioneers in transplantation immunology joined these efforts. The lack for a good proper progression in skin transplantation and the initial encouraging data on experimental renal transplantation shifted the scientific attention from skin and soft tissue transplantation to human renal transplantation, which showed a more promising outcome. In 1954, Joseph Murray performed the first successful renal transplantation in humans between identical twins. Renal transplantation across the MHC followed, with the introduction of azathioprine as immunosuppressive agent. For this achievement, Murray received the Nobel Prize in medicine and physiology, and he remains the only plastic surgeon that has received such honour to date. These pioneering works and efforts were the opening of a new era in transplantation medicine. The evolution of renal transplantation encouraged other solid organ transplantation (SOT) programmes in the last decades of the twentieth century, such as heart, liver, lung, pancreas and small bowel transplants. During the same period, though, there was little progress on the exploration of clinical skin and soft tissue transplantation, most probably by

the conception that skin was one of the most immunogenicity tissues in the human body. The former being reinforced by the pioneering experience of Gilbert in Ecuador, were doctors performed the first-hand transplantation ever in 1964, which was rejected despite the implementation of prednisone and azathioprine immunosuppression. More than 30 years elapsed between this first exploration of VCA and the first successful hand transplantation in 1998. The improvement in immunosuppression regimes and the introduction of new drugs (calcineurin inhibitors, cyclosporine A and tacrolimus, and mycophenolate mofetil) were grounds for improvement in survival (liver, heart, pancreas, lungs) and for the introduction of new SOT programmes such as small bowel transplantation. Their introduction in experimental models showed promising results in VCA in experimental animals. These impressive results prompted authors to organise a research team on human VCA at the University of Louisville, Kentucky, which showed good results in big experimental animals with long-term survival, proving the role of this preclinical study protocol. At the same time, other clinical scientists at the Cleveland Clinic (Strome and co-workers) developed experimental studies on laryngeal transplantation, and Hoffman and co-workers, experimental studies on knee joint transplantation. Few years of research brought these types of transplantations to the clinic. Other teams were formed in Louisville and Lyon, aiming to perform human hand and upper extremity allotransplantation. The first human hand allotransplantation was performed in France (Lyon) in September 1998, followed by the Louisville team in January 1999. All initial efforts helped to the development of the initial VCA teams to date that have made a reality in the human clinic vascularised composite tissue allotransplantation of the hand, larynx, knee, femur, abdominal wall, upper and lower extremities and face (Fig. 1.7).

The initial development of hand allotransplantation programmes helped in the understanding of the performance of immunosuppression protocols, rejection episodes and their treatment and functional and midterm outcomes of VCA. Similarly, the initial outcomes of different VCA programmes have shown that a robust team and VCA protocol and good patient selection allow for excellent clinical results and good survival.

History of Face Transplantation and Objectives

Abstract

The recent history of face transplantation includes a few chronological key issues that promoted the development of face VCA in the past few years. In November 2004, following an increasing scientific, social and mass media interest, the Royal College of Surgeons in London released the "Working Party Report on Face Transplantation", which concluded that at that point further basic science, psychological and translational research was necessary to implement the discipline in human clinical practice. At that moment in time, though, the University of Louisville had published a series of documents pointing out the ethical and scientific relevance of face transplantation in selected patients.

The recent history of face transplantation includes a few chronological key issues that promoted the development of face VCA in the past few years. In November 2004, following an increasing scientific, social and mass media interest, the Royal College of Surgeons in London released the "Working Party Report on Face Transplantation", which concluded that at that point further basic science, psychological and translational research was necessary to implement the discipline in human clinical practice. At that moment in time, though, the University of Louisville had published a series of documents pointing out the ethical and scientific relevance of face transplantation in selected patients.

The same year, the CCNE (Comité Consultatif National d'Ethique) in France was in favour of the implementation in clinical practice of a partial human transplantation, although expressed its reserve for an integral, full-face transplantation. Few months later, in October 2005, the Ethics Committee of the Cleveland Clinic granted permission for a face transplantation to Dr. Siemionow's team (world expert and pioneer in experimental face transplantation) to perform face transplantation in humans. In 2005, the American Society of Plastic Surgery (ASPS) produced a similar document to that of the Royal College of Surgeons in London, serving as a clinical guide, recommending the practice of human face programmes in gradual increments. Soon afterwards, human face transplantation became a reality in Amiens, France, where doctors (Dr. Bernard Devauchelle and Dr. Jean Michel Dubernard) within a multidisciplinary

J.P. Barret, V. Tomasello, *Face Transplantation: Principles, Techniques and Artistry*,
DOI 10.1007/978-3-662-45444-2_2, © Springer-Verlag Berlin Heidelberg 2015

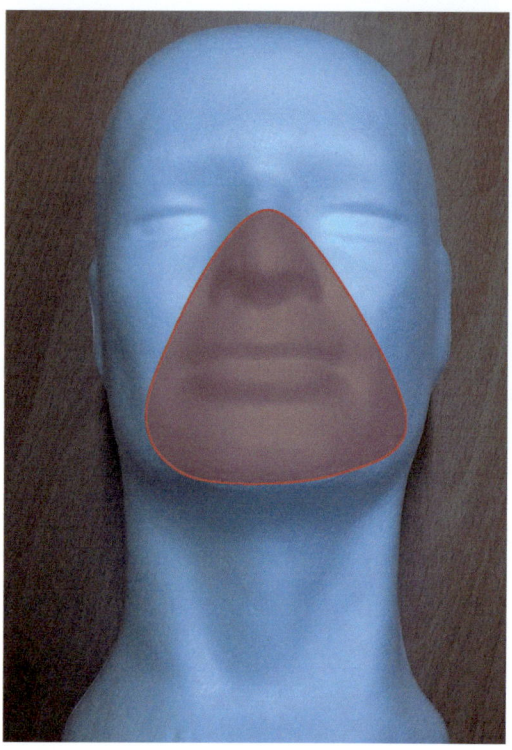

Fig. 2.1 The world's first human face transplantation. The lower third of the face, including the lips and oral commissures, was transplanted

team performed the world's first partial human face transplantation (Fig. 2.1). The intervention was performed on a woman who had suffered the attack of a domestic dog, sustaining the loss of the lower part of her face. Initial and midterm report on the intervention granted the success of the transplantation, followed by good to excellent documentation of sensory and functional recovery. The medical community and society in general had a favourable response to this transplantation. Following this first case, subsequent favourable ethical reports for face transplantation programmes were achieved in the Netherlands (University Hospital Utrecht) and in the UK (Royal Free Hospital, Dr. Peter Butler). At this point in time, a general acceptance was observed on the immunological survival of face transplants, sensory and functional recovery, with a technique far superior to conventional reconstructive surgery.

Few reports on successful face transplantation followed this initial experience. In April

2006, Dr. Shuzhong Guo, at the Xijing Hospital in Xian (China), performed the world's second partial face transplantation in a male patient affected by a traumatic deformity on the lower face caused by a bear's attack. Results were similar to that obtained in the first face transplantation. Other partial face transplantations followed: neurofibromatosis and wound shot injuries to the face in Paris (Dr. Lantieri), wound shot injury to the face in the USA (Dr. Siemionow), electrical burn injury (Boston, Dr. Pomahac) and postoncological deformity and neurofibromatosis in Spain (Valencia, Dr. Cavadas; Seville, Dr. Gomez-Cia). In April 2009, the first partial face and double hand transplantation is attempted (Dr. Lantieri, Paris). Although initially successful, the operation failed few weeks afterwards due to infection and septic shock.

Face transplantation made the final step forward in March 2010. For the first time in the world, the first full face transplantation was performed. The operation was successful, and it resolved many technical, scientific and ethical questions unsolved until that moment. The recipient, a 30-year-old male patient affected by a severe posttraumatic injury from a gunshot injury to the face received a full face transplant (skin, muscle, lips, eyelids, lachrymal apparatus, mucosa, palate, upper and lower teeth, nerves, etc.) that included all face bones (Dr. Barret; Barcelona, Spain). The operation was successful, and the patient regained his premorbid status a few months after his operation. This operation changed the approach to face restoration through face transplantation. From that moment on, face transplantation will be performed following aesthetic units with strict reconstructive tenets. Therefore, full-face transplantation will be performed in those patients affected by severe deformities covering different aesthetic units, reserving partial ones for strict aesthetic units.

Currently, a total of 26 face transplantations have been performed worldwide (France 10, USA 7, Spain 3, China 1, Belgium 1, Turkey 3, Poland 1) covering 13 different institutions in the world.

2.1   Vascularised Composite Tissue Allotransplantation

Face transplantation is a perfect example of composite tissue allotransplantation (CTA), more recently termed as vascularised composite tissue allotransplantation (VCA). The progression in reconstructive surgery has made this type of transplantation reconstruction a reality. Composite tissue allotransplantation began in 1998 in human clinic, when a team performed the first human hand transplantation in France. Following this, other parts of the body, including the abdominal wall, limbs, genitals, tendons, larynx, muscles, nerves, tongue and face, have been attempted throughout the world. This is an emerging subspecialty in the field of transplantation (Fig. 2.1). These VCA are distinct from traditional solid organ transplantations (kidneys, liver, heart, lungs, pancreas); however, they have in common the same tenets of transplantation surgery, namely, the necessity of a vascular pedicle for survival and the requirement for an intense immunosuppression regime to prevent rejection. The former makes an important and relevant difference from allotransplantation of isolated tissues (skin, bones, tendons, etc.), which are used as nonvascularised tissues, being used in clinical practice for many years. Face and hand VCA have been included in an independent classification (Gordon type III) that differs from other types of transplants (Table 2.1), which is based on the surgical complexity and the rehabilitation and psychological impact. Currently, it is accepted that there exist 13 different types of vascularised composite tissue allotransplantation, depending on the combination of tissues, the amount of skin and its antigenicity, making Banff classification a necessity but a lively changing scoring system.

VCA has changed the reconstructive paradigm in plastic and reconstructive surgery. There exist millions of patients with different types of deformities not amenable for a full functional reconstruction with traditional techniques. Common examples are catastrophic deformities to the face (with loss of eyelids, lips, tongue and larynx) and unilateral and bilateral limb amputations. This new field of transplantation has come

Table 2.1 Modified Gordon CTA classification system based on relative complexity

Type	Complexity	Allografts	Characteristics
I	Low	Flexor tendon	1. Absent skin
		Tongue	2. Reduced antigenicity
		Uterus	
		Vascularised nerve	
II	Moderate	Abdominal wall	1. Contain skin
		Face subunit (ear)	2. Absent or less challenging rehabilitation
		Genitalia (penis)	
		Larynx	
		Scalp	
		Trachea	
		Vascularised joint (knee)	
III	High	Upper extremity (hand)	1. Requires multidisciplinary transplant team
		Face	2. Complex rehabilitation
			3. Significant psychological obstacles
			4. Complicate cortical reorganisation
IV	Maximum	Concomitant CTA	1. High mortality risk
		Face/hand(s)	2. Extreme difficulty
		Face/tongue rehabilitation	

From Siemionow M, Zor F, Gordon CR. Face and upper extremity transplantation: future challenges and potential concerns. Plast Reconstr Surg. 2010;126(1):308–15 to reality following an extensive experimental research that has been translated to human clinic. All published data, regarding experimental work, and the human multidisciplinary approach have proven that a robust team approach in a tertiary hospital setting can produce excellent outcomes, which are technically, psychologically and ethically acceptable.

2.2 Objectives in Face Transplantation

Face transplantation is still evolving, being on its initial phases of development worldwide. Therefore, it is still considered a clinical experimental venture. The implication of these considerations is that it is a new technique with unknown long-term results, especially considering its longevity and chronic rejection. Consequently, the indication for face transplantation has to be made on a case-by-case basis by a multidisciplinary team.

Current objectives of face transplantation include:

1. The introduction of a new method of restorative surgery for patients that present with severe catastrophic face deformities, caused by severe burns, trauma, congenital deformities or tumours, having in common the utilisation of microsurgical techniques and plastic

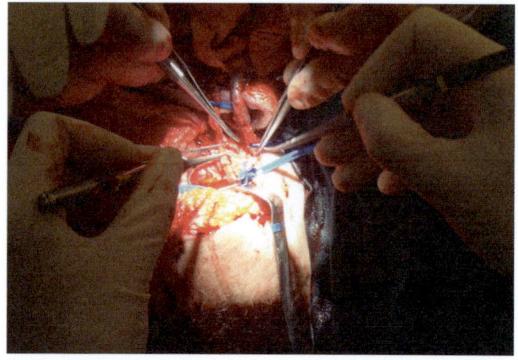

Fig. 2.2 Microsurgical techniques are necessary to perform human face composite tissue allotransplantation

surgery methodology for the transplantation of composite face tissues (Fig. 2.2)
2. To obtain optimal outcomes, both functional psychological and aesthetic, with "restitutio ad integrum" of the deformed structures
3. Optimal reconstruction of the face, with complete restoration of the missing anatomy, not amenable for reconstruction with any other traditional technique(s)
4. To produce the necessary outcomes for the reintegration of the patient into society, family and work market

As in many other areas of plastic surgery, the line between what is desirable, necessary and ethical is very subtle.

Indications for Face Transplantation

3

Abstract

Severe face deformity is one of the most devastating disabilities of human beings. In the majority of cases, this disability produces a myriad of symptoms, including depression, social isolation and suicide ideation. In comparison to other extreme disabilities, such as amputations, spinal cord injuries or cerebrovascular disease, where compassion and sympathy are common reactions in those that relate with the patients and in society in general, catastrophic face deformities produce anxiety, rejection and fear in those that are confronted with them. Physicians that care for this people ordinarily listen to histories of rejection and isolation feelings, fear to expose oneself to society for being "ugly" or "anger gazes" and even increpations such as "how one dares to walk on the street with such a face" or "you are scaring my children".

Severe face deformity is one of the most devastating disabilities of human beings. In the majority of cases, this disability produces a myriad of symptoms, including depression, social isolation and suicide ideation. In comparison to other extreme disabilities, such as amputations, spinal cord injuries or cerebrovascular disease, where compassion and sympathy are common reactions in those that relate with the patients and in society in general, catastrophic face deformities produce anxiety, rejection and fear in those that are confronted with them. Physicians that care for this people ordinarily listen to histories of rejection and isolation feelings, fear to expose oneself to society for being "ugly" or "anger gazes" and even increpations such as "how one dares to walk on the street with such a face" or "you are scaring my children".

Traditional methods of reconstructive plastic surgery include the transplantation of neighbouring tissues to the defect, free tissue transfers and the use of prosthesis and biomaterials. Best outcomes are most often obtained when the surgeon can utilise tissues from adjacent face areas, rendering a good colour and texture match. However, when dealing with severe deformities, these tissues are either absent or injured and deformed also. In these situations, the techniques that are available to reconstruct patients offer outcomes that are far from perfect and do not obtain the desired goal—restoration of image and function—rendering poor quality of life.

J.P. Barret, V. Tomasello, *Face Transplantation: Principles, Techniques and Artistry*,
DOI 10.1007/978-3-662-45444-2_3, © Springer-Verlag Berlin Heidelberg 2015

Reconstruction often fills the defect with tissue, and social appearance is mediocre. Feelings of isolation, rejection, anxiety and depression are not being overcome and maintain a high level of stress and psychological problems. In many instances, patients require a large number of operations to attempt achieving the desired outcome (some cases require more than 100 interventions in a long lifespan), having a final result far from perfect.

Face transplantation is an excellent alternative to traditional treatments for severe and catastrophic face deformities. Its application in selected cases has been a revolution in reconstructive surgery, similar to that achieved with solid organ transplantation for patients with endorgan failure years ago. Paralleling that experience, it is producing the same social demands and it raises similar scientific and ethical questions. The transplantation of face structures permits the reconstruction of disfigured face anatomy with healthy tissues that have a preformed natural form and function, the final outcome being superb in comparison to that yielded by traditional techniques. All scarred and deformed tissues and anatomical landmarks are resected. Following this step, identical, healthy tissues replace them. A normal functional, sensorial and social outcome is expected at 1–2 years. All techniques that are necessary to perform face transplants are commonly used on a daily basis in tertiary plastic surgery services. Among them, the microsurgical proficiency, which permits anastomosing vessels and nerves and joining together muscles and all anatomical structures, is routinely performed. The outcomes of face transplantation programmes throughout the world warrant that with a robust protocol and team approach, these perfect outcomes can be achieved.

3.1 Indications

Face transplantation is in its initial clinical phase. Therefore, it should be still considered a clinical experimental treatment. The effects and long-term outcomes are still unknown; thus, face transplantation should be considered and evaluated on a case-by-case basis. In order to provide the maximum safety of the procedure and achieve equilibrium between the potential risks (including death as an outcome) and the benefits to patients affected by severe face deformities, the indications should be limited and be meticulously defined. As mentioned before, it is evaluated in an individualised manner, and it is limited to true severe face deformities that cannot be properly reconstructed with traditional techniques. Focus on functional outcome is essential.

Absolute indications for face transplantation include:

- Complete destruction of the eyelids, including the orbital sphincter
- Complete destruction of the lips, including the oral muscle sphincter

Destruction of face muscle sphincters cannot be currently restored or reconstructed with traditional techniques. There have been attempts to mimic the natural function of these structures with composite free tissue transfer (free flaps). However, results vary and they are poor, both functionally and aesthetically. Therefore, we may assume that the only and unique technique that can render a total restoration of the face sphincters is the transplantation of such structures from a human being (donor) that granted permission for face transplantation. With this manoeuvre, the delicate muscle, internal lining, nerves, vessels and skin of these anatomical landmarks can be properly reconstructed.

Taking into account the former considerations, diseases and anatomical conditions that constitute absolute indications for face transplantation can be listed (Table 3.1):

1. Patients affected by face destruction (total or partial) from burns
2. Posttraumatic face deformities
3. Benign tumours, congenital deformities and other local extensive malformations

Patients affected by burn squeals present with a broad spectrum of deformity (Figs. 3.1 and 3.2). It may vary from small superficial scarring that produces aesthetic deformities to total destruction of anatomy and function. There have

Table 3.1 Types of general indications for face transplantation

Aetiology	Considerations
Postburn deformity	Evaluate psychosocial impact and functional status; severe scarred faces may not be good indications
Posttraumatic deformities	Important complexity, bone commonly involved; good indication if functional impact is severe. Gunshot injuries are excellent indication
Benign tumours and congenital deformities	Good indications if pan-face deformity is present. May require treatment of tumour/malformation first, followed by transplantation. Neurofibromatosis and AV malformations excellent indications
Postoncological deformities	Severe deformities. Evaluate on a case-by-case with oncology. Check oncological risk and functional impact
	Important ethical issues

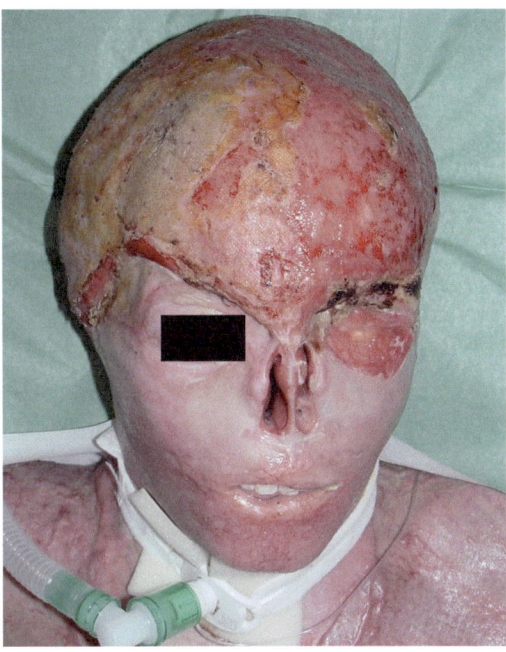

Fig. 3.2 Destruction of face sphincters and severe face scarring are common problems in burn patients that have an indication for face VCA

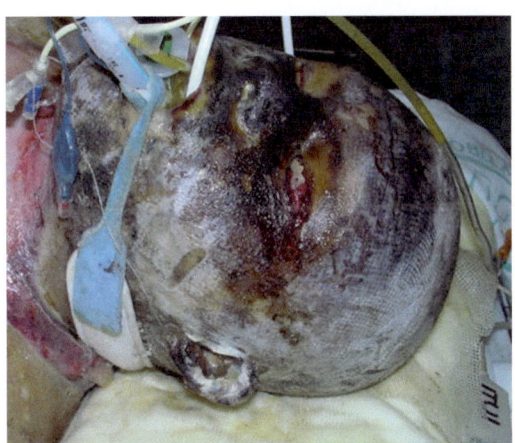

Fig. 3.1 Massive third-degree burns to the face are good candidates for face VCA. It may be considered in the acute phase for patients with the involvement of deep structures

been diverse face transplantations on burn patients, all having in common destruction of oral and/or eyelid sphincters. Postburn pan-face deformity should be addressed with caution, especially in those patients with scarred faces with minimal functional deficits. In this patient population though, deformities may pose significant psychological and social impact. The indication should be carefully addressed on a case-by-case basis, taking into consideration the risk–benefit of the procedure.

Posttraumatic face deformity (Figs. 3.3 and 3.4) is a second important group of patients that may benefit from face transplantation. Deformities of the soft tissues are commonly encountered, coupled with bony destruction and functional incompetence. Gunshots to the face are a paradigm of such deformities. The latter are formal indications for face transplantation. Similar to burn deformity, the patient should be thoroughly evaluated. Some patients function well in society and face transplantation may not be indicated in these situations.

Benign tumours and congenital/acquired malformations are commonly treated in tertiary plastic surgery departments (Figs. 3.5 and 3.6). Most of them are treated within a multidisciplinary team with good to excellent outcomes. Patients present with localised or restricted tumours/

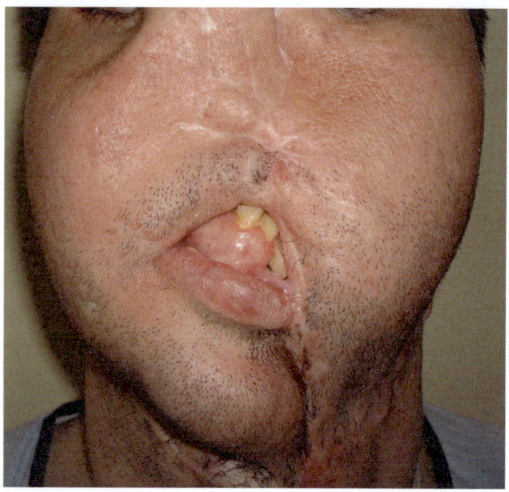

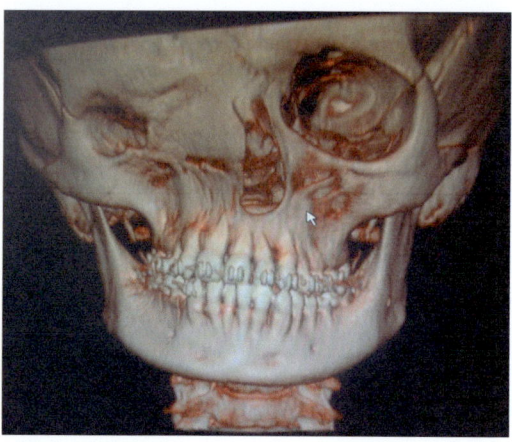

Fig. 3.5 Complex congenital deformities may benefit from a face VCA team approach, which is aimed to reconstruct face sphincters and anatomical landmarks and face bones

Fig. 3.3 Gunshot injuries to the face are excellent indication for face transplantation. They allow for immediate restoration of form and function

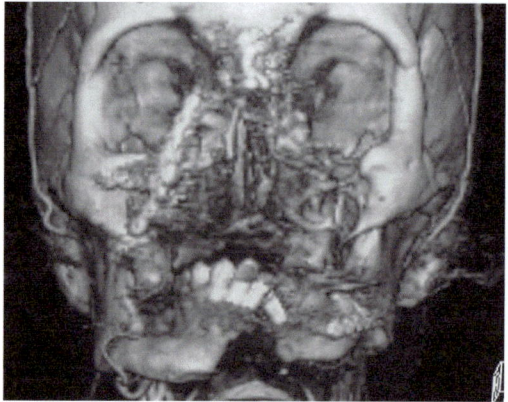

Fig. 3.4 Posttraumatic bone involvement can be restored with a composite tissue face allotransplantation that includes the maxilla and the mandible

deformities, and traditional or classical techniques after formal resection of the cause of the deformity render acceptable functional and aesthetic results. Large and severe tumours/deformities require multiple operations and mutilations. Consequently, patients required a long-term follow-up, a large number of operations, difficult rehabilitation and a secondary deformity (both aesthetic and functional) caused by the surgical treatment. This kind of patient reintegrates badly into society and function is commonly impaired. These types of patients are good

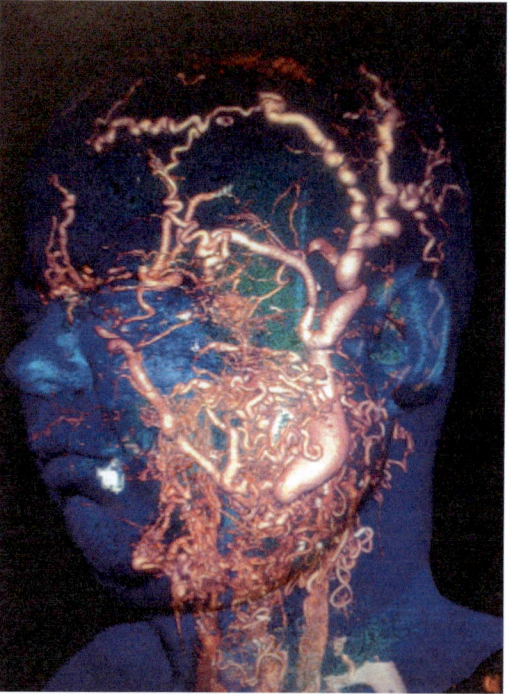

Fig. 3.6 Vascular malformations and neurofibromatosis are also prime indications in face VCA programmes. They allow resection of the tumour and restoration of anatomy

candidates for face transplantation, provided they understand the nature of the treatment, its limitations and the potential and real risks. Common

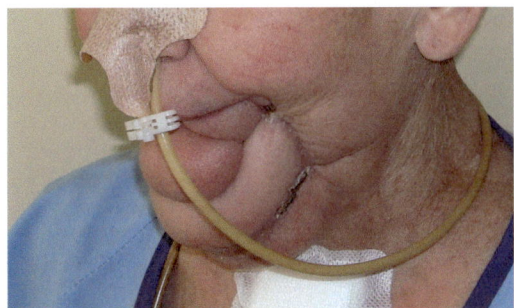

Fig. 3.7 Postoncological deformities should be evaluated in a case-by-case basis with full oncology work-up to rule out other primaries, recurrences and the individual oncological risk

aetiologies include type I neurofibromatosis, vascular malformation and secondary craniofacial deformities.

Postoncological deformities deserve a special word of caution (Fig. 3.7). They are common, especially in large tertiary care centres. Their aesthetic and functional impact is severe, although their unique biology deserves an individualised approach. Even though they are not formal contraindications for face transplantation, it is well accepted that immunosuppression can promote the development of recurrences or newly acquired cancer tumours from silent clones of cancer cells. The experimental nature of face transplantation limits its utilisation in this patient population. If they are to be evaluated, patients should be "cured" from their disease and follow a complete check-up by the oncology department. The oncological risk of the patient has to be evaluated and a final decision be made. It has to be remembered that almost all patients affected by oncological deformities have received preoperative or postoperative radiotherapy, causing an added deformity and defect in tissues, with extensive fibrosis that may prevent transplants to be functionally correct.

3.1.1 Contraindications for Face Transplantation

A list of indications and contraindications for face transplantation may produce an intense

debate, similar to that produced in society during the first four years of the twenty-first century regarding face transplantation.

Contraindications for face transplantation vary with time, centre, culture and country. They must be listed in the face transplant protocol, and they usually follow a consensus with the ethical committee and the transplant organisation body of the region/country. In general terms, however, we may accept that the following are absolute contraindications for face transplantation:

1. Evidence of tumour malignancy
2. Negative report from psychiatric/psychological evaluation (active psychiatric disorders, severe personality disorders and known and reported non-compliance to treatments, among others)
3. Medical conditions that affect systems and/or organs (especially those that may be affected by immunosuppression drugs)

3.1.2 The Timing for Face Transplantation

The initial approach and formulation of clinical protocols indicated that face VCA was an experimental clinical treatment that should only be attempted in cases with no other alternatives and as a last resort. Indeed, long-term outcomes were still unknown, and the efficacy of face transplantation for restoration of form and function in an effective manner had to be explored. However, the indication of a face transplantation under these circumstances raises important ethical questions.

Obtaining informed consent when nothing else can be offered as a method of treatment makes informed consent almost impossible. Without a reasonable alternative, patients cannot counterbalance risks and benefits of different techniques and approaches for the deformity, and this increases the stress and the inability to make plausible decisions. Moreover, clinical protocols stated that there should be an alternative to reconstruct the defect should the transplant failed and return the patient to the premorbid condition. Even though this is a formal requirement for ethical accreditation, it would be almost impossible to return patients to the pre-transplant appearance and function if no other alternatives are possible. On the other hand, this line of treatment would condemn patients to a large number of unnecessary operations when reconstruction of a severe deformity is performed with traditional techniques: the final outcome will be less than acceptable, and the patients will be then confronted with the difficult decision to accept a face VCA as a last resort.

The evolution of the successful team approach for face transplantation and the good to excellent outcomes that have been obtained forced this approach to be turned to a more aggressive and early indication for face transplantation.

It is our belief, which is shared by others, that patients with complex and severe face deformities that cannot be reconstructed with traditional techniques be offered a face VCA early in the treatment plan process. All other donor sites and techniques will be still available should the transplant failed, and the patient will show less scarring, untouched face tissues and good alternatives for acceptor vessels and nerves. The evolution of face transplantation in its early stages has rapidly

Table 3.2 Timing of face VCA indication

	Positive effects	Negative effects
Early	Avoids unnecessary operations	Halts reconstructive plan
	Limits scarring	Increases time in waiting list with functional problems
	Preserves vessels and nerves	Limits acceptance of functional deficits
	Low stress level	
	Limits transfusions and immunological barriers	
Late	Better acceptance of functional deficits	Limits rescue operations
	Allows good communication with team and surgeons	Large number of operations
	Increases patient compliance	Increases scarring
		Acceptor vessels and nerves may be limited
		Ethical problems in informed consent

changed to a more restorative surgery, changing the paradigm of face reconstruction and face transplantation (Table 3.2).

Psychological, Social and Ethical Issues

4

Abstract

The success of face transplantation throughout the world has positioned this technique as a new option for patients presenting with severe face deformities. However, the transplantation of a cadaver's donor face still poses important psychological, social and ethical issues into the medical community. Current consensus advises doctors to evaluate potential candidates within a multidisciplinary team in a tertiary centre performing solid organ transplantation on a daily basis. Core members of such multidisciplinary team include plastic surgeons, immunologists, infectious diseases specialists, psychiatrists, psychologists, transplant surgeons, transplant coordinators, rehabilitation specialists and social workers, among others.

4.1 Psychosocial and Ethical Considerations of Face Transplantation

The success of face transplantation throughout the world has positioned this technique as a new option for patients presenting with severe face deformities. However, the transplantation of a cadaver's donor face still poses important psychological, social and ethical issues into the medical community. Current consensus advises doctors to evaluate potential candidates within a multidisciplinary team in a tertiary centre performing solid organ transplantation on a daily basis. Core members of such multidisciplinary team include plastic surgeons, immunologists, infectious diseases specialists, psychiatrists, psychologists, transplant surgeons, transplant coordinators, rehabilitation specialists and social workers, among others.

A decade ago, Siemionow and Ogich pointed out that patients affected from severe face deformity would improve dramatically their quality of life with face transplantation. Thus, they signalled that patient should be involved in the decision-making process of face transplantation. Still, in 2004 the French National Ethics Advisory Committee affirmed that it was too soon for face transplantation accreditation and did not grant permission for total face transplantation, since they considered that the discipline could not answer positively the risk–benefit ratio dilemma. In November 2005, though, the same French committee granted permission for the first partial human transplantation. Organ transplantation carries with it a series of psychosocial problems. They are exacerbated in the case of

J.P. Barret, V. Tomasello, *Face Transplantation: Principles, Techniques and Artistry*,
DOI 10.1007/978-3-662-45444-2_4, © Springer-Verlag Berlin Heidelberg 2015

Table 4.1 Requirements for face VCA

1. Centre with proven solid organ transplantation experience
2. Tertiary/university centre with all clinical and research services on site
3. Plastic surgery department with proven experience in microsurgery and craniomaxillofacial surgery
4. VCA team
5. Face transplant VCA protocol approved by the Ethics Committee
6. Accreditation by transplantation bodies and organ procurement organisations

Table 4.2 Psychological response to face transplantation

Fear for transplant failure
Fear for rejection episodes
Anxiety regarding side effects and complications
Self-responsibility on the success of the transplant
Treatment adherence
Feeling ill (becoming chronic patient)
Integration in self-image
Emotional response regarding donors
Questions of identity and communication
Personal adaptation to deformity

face transplantation, specially for questions of identity, communication, psychological vulnerability, the aesthetic results, possibility of death, treatment compliance and the patient's and relatives' reaction to a new identity. These are scientific and ethical issues that need to be addressed by any face transplantation protocol. The first human transplantation protocol approved ever by an Ethics or IRB Committee occurred in 2004 in the Cleveland Clinic (Dr. Siemionow, USA). The accreditation of a human protocol must include the inclusion and exclusion criteria, patients' screening, informed consents for recipients and donors and the multidisciplinary team to develop the programme (Table 4.1). Only under theses auspices—the "face transplant protocol"—patients with severe face deformity may be evaluated for face transplantation indication.

4.2 Psychological and Social Aspects of Transplantation

4.2.1 The Psychological Response

The development of organ transplantation programmes has had an important effect on the research for the human psychological response and adaptation in recipients. It has been traditionally accepted that organ transplantation can produce a series of stressing factors and may trigger a change in the psychosocial adaptation. They include:

- The longevity of the graft (fear for transplanted organ failure)
- Fear for rejection episodes

- Long-term anxiety regarding the potential side effects of transplantation immunosuppression protocols, including viral infections and malignant tumours
- The personal responsibility on the success or failure of the transplanted tissue/organ: medication regime adherence/compliance, changing social lifestyle, monitoring signs and symptoms, the chronic dependence to an ambulatory setting ("feeling ill")
- The integration of the transplant in self-image and self-identity
- The emotional response related to organ transplantation (receiving a transplanted organ; guilt feelings, specially related to donor and donor's relatives)

When we consider face transplantation separately, all these fears, guilt feelings, anxiety, etc. are amplified (Table 4.2). Reasons for this behaviour include questions of identity and communication, personal psychological adaptation to deformity and support.

4.2.2 Identity and Communication

Our face is extremely relevant for the development and maintenance of our identity. It helps us and others to understand ourselves, our whereabouts, who we are and our prospects. If we are deprived of a face, we can no longer recognise ourselves; our body image disaggregates, causing a profound existential crisis. We may follow, thus, that introducing a new face (that of the others, the donor) may bring problems even worse than those pre-existing, especially in the area of identity.

Conscious and unconscious face expressions are necessary to relate and communicate with the rest of the world. One-third of the communication with other people is non-verbal, depending on face expressions. The coordination of face muscles, nerves and tissues is essential for this part of human interaction. There are different pathways that connect face structures and cerebral functioning, recognising our status of expression, i.e. smiling signals neuronal connections that in turn produce a feeling of well-being. More research will be necessary to understand how the face mimic influences our psychological status.

4.2.3   Psychological Adaptation to Deformity

It is well supported in literature that psychological stress is not necessarily proportional to the severity of face deformity. Some patients function well with severe devastating injuries, whereas others show important stress and anxiety with small scars and minimal deformities. When we consider trauma patients, it is not uncommon to diagnose important levels of stress and anxiety, although it is not per se a formal indication for transplantation. The same patient may show excellent psychosocial adaptation in the rehabilitation and chronic phase. However, we may not assume, though, that time is a good remedy for face deformity adaptation. Patients that adapt well have in common a high threshold of self-esteem, good family and social support, excellent communication skills and a sense that the deprivation of a normal face should not impede happiness and good quality of life. On the other hand, patients that show difficulties in social adaptation believe that physical appearance is of paramount importance for well-being and success. They show important levels of anxiety, depression and psychosocial difficulties, searching surgery to improve physical appearance and improve their social interaction and sense of well-being. In general terms, this group of patients is psychologically very vulnerable, although they show a

high motivation for surgery and compliance. Still, non-realistic expectations regarding surgical outcomes may be present. They require strong team support since they are very vulnerable during the postoperative period, specially regarding uncertainty of final outcomes and treatment side effects. When we deal with this type of patients, it is imperative to follow them closely. We understand that some of our treatments do not offer a complete resolution of symptoms, and secondary deformities may be present. It is also uncertain whether the salutary effects of face transplants, particularly in the sphere of psychosocial improvement and social interaction, will be maintained over time.

4.2.4   Psychological Support for Face Transplant Patients

A good psychological support is essential throughout the whole process of face transplantation for recipients, family members and donor's family and relatives. Specialised professionals well versed in face deformity and solid organ transplantation should perform it. Psychiatrists and psychologists are core members of the face transplant team, dealing with:

- Validation of face transplant recipients; a negative report contraindicates face transplantation.
- Understanding risks and benefits of the proposed treatment.
- Therapeutic support during the search for donors.
- Therapeutic support during the post-operative period and long-term support.
- Recipient's family support during the whole process of transplantation.
- If necessary, donor's family therapeutic support.

4.2.4.1   Validation of Face Transplantation Patients
Motivation and the Patient's Expectations
Patient's journey through a face transplantation treatment process is not an easy one. A long waiting time during the search for donors should be

Table 4.3 Validation of face transplantation patients

1. Evaluate patient's motivation and expectations
2. Past treatment adhesion (patient's compliance)
3. Communication issues and quality of life
4. Explore family and social support
5. Psychological and psychiatric issues

expected, coupled with a high stress level focused on the expectation of a complex operation, the possibility of complications and side effects, the adaptation to a new identity and the possibility of rejection and even death. Patients' expectations are usually very high; they present with important aesthetic and functional deformities, and many of them have gone through other plastic surgery interventions. The face transplant team must understand completely all issues and problems that motivated the patient to search for a face transplantation, address them and create a treatment master plan that can deal with the deformity and all functional problems (Table 4.3). It is very important to address non-realistic expectations in the preoperative period; failure to do so may deal to important postoperative problems, specially with issues of patient compliance with treatments and immunosuppression protocol drugs, psychological adaptation, adhesion to rehabilitation programme and final functional outcome.

The majority of patients will show different levels of anxiety in the area of resilience and the confrontation with the unknown, the possibility of side effects and complications and the new identity. They must be thoroughly evaluated and reassured when necessary to be able to go through the period of search for donors.

Face transplantation is a non-saving procedure; in other terms, the operation is aimed to increase quality of life. Comparing to solid organ transplantation, it mimics renal transplantation; it is performed to improve the life of patients, stop dialysis and provide patients with a long-term superior treatment. However, when dealing with risks and possible outcomes, we can compare it to heart transplantation: should the transplant failed, only a new transplant could solve the problem. Ultimately, death can be the outcome. Consequently, a good cognitive level is necessary

to understand the risks and the benefits of the proposed treatment. Good motivated patients should be assessed by the transplant team and evaluated that the patient understands that the possible benefits and the potential improvement in quality of life surpasses the potential risks and that patient accepts them as part of the treatment. The expected improvement in quality of life and the manner the patient feels and accepts it should be superior to the potential morbidity and mortality.

4.3　Protocol Adhesion, Preoperative and Postoperative Support

Good adhesion and patient's compliance with the postoperative protocol is necessary for the success of face transplantation. When we compare data regarding other type of solid organ transplantation, it is reported that as much as 46 % of recipients of solid organ transplants do not adhere to the postoperative protocol. In order to make an approximation to the patient's own risk of protocol non-adhesion, team members evaluate the past medical history and the patient's adhesion to clinic visits and other types of treatment protocols followed in the past. Patient's behaviours reflecting clinic no-shows, failure to perform treatments and tests and stopping at own risk medications are red flags that need to be addressed. It is indeed a complex interaction of different factors, including personal and cultural characteristics, education level, understanding instructions and the intrinsic complexity of the treatment. They will signal future adhesion to the transplantation protocol, including in these considerations the familiar and social support, which are also important pillars in patient's compliance. On the other hand, it is relevant to assess the capacity of patients for changing the environment and different lifestyles: it is not uncommon that after the transplant, sun exposure may be limited, housing may be required to be changed, and pets may not be allowed. We should remember that many patients may enter the face transplantation programme, but only few may have a

Table 4.4 Special issues that complicate social and personal adaptation in the postoperative period

Communication problems (oral impairment, tracheotomy)
Face paralysis
Feeding problems
Sensory recovery
Reactions of others
Mass media interest

true indication for a face transplant. Tertiary centres are best positioned to offer patients with face disfigurement psychological support and all types of treatment options. Those that do not fulfil all requirements for face transplantations have to be followed, supported and offered other reconstructive treatment options if they are indicated.

Patients that have been accredited as potential candidates and that have a true indication for transplantation enter the programme. It is not uncommon that patients have to wait a long time during the search for donors. During this period a good support and periodical visits to the team members are fundamental. Support is delivered constantly and reinforced when needed. During this period the patient's expectations are readdressed, and different issues regarding the intraoperative and postoperative period are reviewed.

During the postoperative period, care has to be implemented to detect any sign of stress, anxiety and/or depression. Patients are normally highly motivated and have been prepared to the postoperative journey. However, communication problems (oral impairment, tracheotomy), difficulties moving the newly acquired face (postoperative face paralysis), feeding problems, etc. may pose an important challenge to the patient. In this phase the team should pay attention to all signs and symptoms for psychological adaptation (Table 4.4). One of the most relevant signs is the adaptation to the new identity, watching the new appearance in the mirror and its acceptance. In general terms, patients should be allowed to see his/her new face as soon as the patient requests to do so. The general response to all face transplants so far is a positive reaction, since patients accept their new reality as new human beings, regardless of the true appearance (they feel normal again).

Following this event, the new self-image is rapidly integrated in the imagination and, in the cerebral plasticity, soon forgetting the deformed face appearance. Patients then remember two selves, the one prior to the deformity and the new identity. Patients that present with congenital deformities or benign tumours (i.e. neurofibromatosis) feel confident and normal for the first time in their life.

Patients are soon requested to take care of the face, to massage scars, to touch the new face and to work together with rehabilitation services; all these manoeuvres help to integrate the new face rapidly. Questions, curiosities and gratitude regarding donors may be necessary to be addressed during this phase of recovery. At the final part of the admission to hospital, the team has to address the programme of gradual social reintegration into society. Other issues that may arise are society and mass media interest-communication. We have to remember that face transplantation is aimed to improve quality of life, its main goal being to reintegrate into society patients with face disfigurement as full active members.

4.4 Life Following Hospital Discharge

4.4.1 Living with a New Appearance

Patients that go through a programme of face transplantation experience three different phases (Table 4.5). Firstly, patients are evaluated; an indication is performed and will go through a long time waiting for a donor search. As soon as the face transplant is a reality, patients are admitted to the hospital and have a hospital stay that may last a few weeks depending on the complexity of the transplants and the potential complications. During this phase the patient is coached and supported, creating a protective environment. Finally, the recipient is discharged from hospital; this final phase may produce new feelings of stress and anxiety. Patients will return to their normal environment and family and social circle; they will be exposed to family and friends'

Table 4.5 Phases of face transplantation

1. Evaluation, indication and search for donors
2. Transplantation and hospital stay, new identity
3. Return to normal environment (family and social)

Table 4.6 Basis for a good indication

1. Inform patients
2. Important deformities
3. Severe impact on quality of life
4. Reasonable cognitive and educational level

reactions, both to their new appearance and their new communication skills. This uncertainty will mark also the future success of the face transplant. It will be necessary to have a constant support for the patient and family. The patient needs to understand that the team's support is ready and can be obtained in a rapid manner anytime during this period. It is not only a question of the new face appearance acceptance, but also to face and learn strategies to control emotions and the new relationship with others. Face sensibility and function will improve constantly during the first year, changing gradually the communication skills and the way the patient relates with people. If mass media has been involved or press releases performed, the patient may be recognised by strangers and attract attention. This situation can be positive for some patients, although may be distressing for others, requiring attention and modulation.

4.4.2 Adhesion to Medical Treatment

Postoperative protocols are very complex, including not only relevant medication protocols (immunosuppression, infection control, medications for side effects) but also rehabilitation and nutritional protocols. Most of the patients adhere to without many problems, not surprising considering they are treated within a robust transplant protocol. Patients that have presented with adhesion problems to the immunosuppression protocol have shown important psychological stress, being the main cause for bad compliance. If this is the case, it is imperative to work with the patient and family members to achieve the psychological well-being and promote good medical adhesion. During this period, patients will be also assessed regarding immunosuppression response and related risk for infections and

cancer development. Depending on the individual risk, different adjustments in drug combinations and drug levels will be necessary. These medical manoeuvres should be explained in a comprehensive and understandable manner to the patient (many of them will have been discussed in the preoperative period) in order to maintain the psychological stability not producing increased levels of stress and anxiety.

4.4.3 The Risk of Rejection and Transplant Failure

Good indications are based on informed patients with important deformities with severe impact on quality of life with a reasonable cognitive and educational level. It cannot be overstated that it is the basis for success in composite tissue allotransplantation (Table 4.6). Acute rejection has been reported in as much as 85 % of all vascularised composite tissue allotransplantation. Patients must be instructed in transplant inspection and control of possible complications. They are an important part of postoperative control protocols. Patients are actively involved, and it can be another source of anxiety and fear. Acute chronic episodes require prompt treatment and hospital admissions, and these repeated episodes of inflammation might produce in turn an increase of fibrosis and deterioration of form and function. The face could become a rigid mask, having an important impact in recipients and in the overall transplant programme evolution. These fears and anxieties are shared with professionals, which, on the other hand, may have a salutary effect on the coaching and support of recipients. In addition, rejection episodes require changes and an increase in immunosuppression drugs. Side effects may be present, and patients should be properly monitored for pathophysiological and psychological impacts.

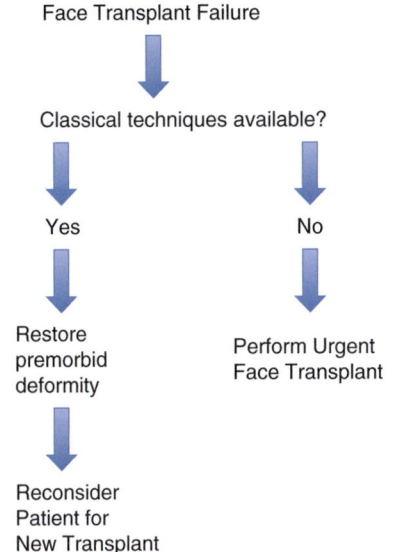

Fig. 4.1   Treatment algorithm in face transplant failure

Similarly to the evolution and fate of solid organ transplantations, transplant failure may occur. Recipients are aware of this potential fatal complication, and it is part of the specific informed consent for face transplantation. If total failure occurs, the face must be removed. This potential complication would cause a significant psychological impact in recipients, family members and transplant team members. It may be possible to proceed at that moment with classical reconstructive techniques (with all its inherent limitations); however, face transplantation has been compared to lung, liver or heart transplantation: failure of the transplant organ can be overcome only with a new transplantation. In general terms, if traditional techniques are possible, the patient would return to its pre-transplant condition (going back to step 1), making a new transplant even more risky (less salvage procedures would be available if a new transplant is attempted). If patients were re-transplanted (bear in mind the shortage of available donors), the patient would go back to a long waiting time and would go through the whole transplant process. In both situations, the psychological support the recipient would require is even more intense than in the primary transplantation (Fig. 4.1).

4.4.4   Effect on Family Members

There has been not much research on the effect of face transplantation on patients' and donor's family members. The most common areas of psychological stress concentrate in:

- There is a high level of responsibility regarding the optimization of the domestic environment and the risk of infection and the maintenance of well-being and health status after the transplant.
- Family members' fears and worries for the future physical and psychological recipient's well-being. There is an important and intense interaction of relatives during the immediate postoperative period, although it tends to diminish gradually months and years after the transplant. On the overall, patients regain a normal social and family status and interaction, going back to a more normal relationship.

The social and psychological intervention should focus, before the transplant, in different areas to warrant the success of the process:

1. Understand the risks and the information to allow complete success
2. Alleviate the stress that family members go through after the patient has made a final decision to accept the procedure and during the search for donors
3. Detect and intervene in the worries regarding future recipient health and psychological status
4. Explore the possible impact that the transplant may pose on relatives and in the social circle of the recipient

During the postoperative period, all family members should be followed and supported to detect pathological levels of stress and anxiety resulting from aesthetic results and functional deficits and false ideations of failures and bad results: encouraging the accent of progressive integration of body image, maintaining immunosuppression protocol, detecting any side effects and promoting emotional experimentation. In case of a transplant failure, psychological family support should be as important and intense as that delivered to the recipient.

The support that the transplant team, and specially transplant coordinators, must deliver to donors' family cannot be overstated. The decision to donate face tissues, when a sudden death from a relative has occurred, carries with it an intense psychological stress. Donating a face brings false but real ideas of identity transplantation. Social and cultural beliefs are extremely diverse, and presentation of the cadaver after donation is no longer possible. Full support to relatives while in the intensive therapy unit (ITU) (the only possible environment were mourning with the in-love will be possible) is mandatory. The whole process of tissue donation is much more complex than in any other solid organ; coordinators have to preserve the normal and correct donation of internal organs (aimed to life-saving procedures) while allowing successful donation of composite vascularised tissues. Mass media relations and journalists and social interests have to be dealt with, since they are often involved. Preservation of anonymity is a must, and even in those prone to celebrity, it should be discouraged to preserve the normal donation process. This type of social issues does apply to recipients and their families. There exists an important social interest in face transplantation, and it is necessary to prepare them for an important impact to their lives soon after the transplantation. Even though an intense stress from mass media can produce anxiety and psychological problems, a well-maintained and delivered relationship and support may bring salutary effects, such as support from anonymous people and a sense of global support. In general terms, society in general understands the real intention of face transplantation: provide patients with a correct quality of life, reintegration to daily normal activities and reintegration into society. Moreover, publicity will improve the idea that a good quality of life is very relevant for patients with severe face disability and that face transplantation may render this complete outcome and will help many patients to come forward and be helped in specialised reconstructive centres.

Table 4.7 Legal issues in face VCA

1. Informed consent and patient autonomy
2. Physician's autonomy
3. Acceptable risk–benefit ratio
4. Collaborative autonomy
5. Death as an outcome
6. Second opinions
7. Experimental consideration of face VCA
8. Define moral, ethical and legal issues
9. Legal issues of donation: double affirmative answer

4.4.5 Ethical and Legal Issues in Face Transplantation

Patients' informed consent is necessary and a legally bounding document and process that is necessary for every single medical and surgical procedure. The patient is the person responsible for the decision to perform surgery, accept the results and consequences of such decision and the risks of the operation. The surgeon plays a player's role provided patients are informed correctly and that the surgical procedure was performed properly and according to accepted standard clinical practice. The surgeon is responsible for the procedure and its good performance and that any change in the accepted procedure is done in the best benefit of the patient. Best performances are obtained when a good collaboration is obtained between the patient and the surgeon, including all collaborators and team members (Table 4.7). The surgical team must maintain patient's autonomy (inform and accept patients decisions), which is more important and superior to the decision to operate and the surgical procedure itself. However, patient's autonomy is not absolute. Patient's decisions and wishes to go through a surgical procedure may have severe risks. Composite tissue allotransplantation carries significant risks, such as immunological rejection (acute and chronic) and drug-related side effects. Most patients accept these risks to obtain the desired quality of life, even when risks are very high and the possible side effects are considerable. Still, the risk–benefit ratio of patient's decisions and the desire and possible results of the operation should be acceptable for the surgeon. The medical team is not obliged whatsoever to follow and perform a surgical intervention unless they are convinced that the outcomes and results are superior to the potential risks and possible complications and they are proportionate. Autonomy, therefore, has to be universal (apply to all parties, patients and medical teams, surgeons) and, in general and optimal terms, be collaborative. It is anticipated that there may be conflicts when patients consider surgeries appropriate and surgeons not and, conversely, situations that confront the desire of surgeons to perform treatments that are not accepted by patients, despite being in their best interests. Face transplantation procedures focus on a difficult issue, since there are clinical situations that, in terms of quality of life, are worse than being dead. The final outcome of face transplantation may be death; therefore, in such situations the autonomy, obtaining informed consent, and developing a collaborative action may be disperse and difficult. Professional consensus should be sought, and in conflicting situations the patients or surgeons may consider a second opinion to help in the decision process and make sure that patient's best interests, life and health are prioritised. This potential conflict is of particular relevance in face transplantation. There is a clear consensus on the devastating impact that severe face disfigurement produces on a human being; hence, the desire for a procedure that aims to improve quality of life is sustained in ethical grounds. However, similarly to other traditional techniques, surgeons may still face a bioethical and professional problem, specially for such procedures that improve the quality of life but that present with an uncertain positive risk–benefit ratio. The conflict may even worsen with the experimental consideration of face transplantation. All uncertainties in face transplantation will stress all patient–surgeon relationships and will challenge a correct decision-making process. In order to achieve a fluent communication and a correct evaluation of patients, teams and centres should define moral and ethical limits and legal issues in a general consensus in all terms of clinical surgical practice and clinical research.

Ethical and legal issues are also of extreme relevance in the donation process. Teams must be well versed in local legal laws and bills in order to proceed under correct accepted pathways. Legal issues vary in every country. However, there is a common general consensus that a double affirmative answer is advised by many in order to proceed with the procurement of composite vascularised allografts: the will of the donor and the will of the relatives, following the Human Tissue Act (2004). A specific informed consent should be provided and as many interviews as necessary should be performed to achieve excellency and compassion during the process. Minimal information that should be provided includes:

- Amount of tissues to be removed and the probable consequences to the donor's aspect
- How tissues will be transplanted to the recipient and the potential benefits of such transplant
- Address identity issues (how similar/different donor–recipient will show after the transplant)
- Mass media and publicity issues

In addition to all direct and indirect issues, problems and considerations listed above, patients, recipients' relatives and donors' relatives should be informed, and they must understand the experimental character of vascularised composite tissue allotransplantation. Surgeons have to understand the risks, benefits and side effects of this treatment in order to be able to inform patients and their families properly. They have the obligation to deliver the information that the transplant team proposes them a new innovative clinical experimental treatment. Consequently, full details regarding current knowledge of face vascularised composite tissue allotransplantation, the absence of long-term results so far, the uncompleted scientific background regarding any experimental treatment and the acceptance of such limited knowledge should be understood and accepted by patients and team members. Many medical and surgical issues are still being studied and discovered, and since many ethical questions arise and we consider a true clinical experimental work, submission of clinical protocols, indications and proposed cases to Ethics Committees is mandatory.

4.5 The Role of Ethics Committee in Patient's Protection

The Research Ethics Committee (REC) or Institutional Review Board (IRB) in the USA has the mandate to warrant that any proposed research study conforms to the ethics recognised in the Helsinki Declaration (Table 4.8). REC examines the research protocol and shall accept it if it protects the dignity, the legal rights, the clinical safety and the well-being of all individuals participating in clinical research. It will allow participation in clinical research provided patients have received all information and they have been offered the opportunity to express all their concerns and all questions have been properly answered in a timely fashion that allows unrushed decisions.

Some patients are extremely fragile and/or vulnerable, therefore may be prone to give informed consent in situations where there exists an important risk. It can be evaluated in situations with a severe disease and an intense doctor–patient relationship. The committee will evaluate these issues and will supervise that researches did not underestimate the risks and overestimate the benefits of the proposed treatment. Particular care is devoted to evaluate and examine the informed consent and the patient's information document in order to provide patients with sufficient information in clear and understandable wording that shall allow a correct decision-making process. Article 22 of the Helsinki Declaration clearly states that anyone accepting to participate in clinical research must

Table 4.8 Ethics committee role in VCA

1. Warrant that protocols follow the Helsinki Declaration
Dignity protection
Maintenance of legal rights
Warrants clinical safety and well-being
2. Protocol provides all relevant information to patients
3. Informed consent
4. Risks–benefits and current clinical knowledge
5. Independence
6. Death as an outcome: review on a case-by-case individual fashion

be properly informed and researchers have to make sure that they have properly understood all information.

Risks–benefits of any clinical experimental research or assay must be rationale and well supported by the clinical protocol and the current clinical knowledge. Any proposed clinical trial aimed to a fragile or vulnerable patient may only be conducted if it responds to their health needs and be beneficial to the health status of the community in general. Benefits should surpass risks, especially when it is related to the condition being investigated. Risk–benefit assessment is very uncertain, especially when taking into consideration minorities and rare diseases. Ethical decisions of RECs are based on their competency, professionalism and in some instances by consultation with related experts. Patients and/or surgeons may disagree with some decisions that do not permit the implementation of the experimental protocol into practice. Still, only those protocols that receive a positive response and accreditation of the local REC may be implemented. Proposed experimental protocols of composite tissue allotransplantation carry with it an important risk, making RECs' mandate very difficult. However, the Helsinki Declaration offers a path for deliberation in these situations. When one considers a disease or health condition that renders death as an outcome or significant or total disabilities, RECs have a much more flexibility to evaluate the risk–benefit of the proposed treatment. The same declaration allows physicians to contemplate experimental treatments when traditional or classical accepted techniques of protocols cannot be efficacious, provided a full informed consent has been obtained. Following the application of these experimental protocols, the efficacy of such treatments and their risk–benefit will be evaluated.

Taking into consideration the level of difficulty that some proposed experimental research protocols pose to the Ethics Committee, it is essential that all RECs be independent. No doubt, every institution that organised itself not only as a clinical health provider but also as a research institute or foundation is obliged by law to host a local Ethics Committee. However, it must be totally independent from any of the institutions that form the local research environment. Their ruling is only effective for that given institution. Any multicenter clinical trial must be submitted individually to each of the ethics committee forming the research team.

Ethics Committees considering face transplant protocols and patient's indications should evaluate different aspects regarding the physical and psychological risks of the technique:

- It is considered a true experimental clinical research.
- Risks, side effects and consequences of face transplantation can be very severe and devastating.
- Physical and psychological risks and impacts are extremely high.

All these factors and the previous consideration are taken into account to deliver proper answers to researchers. In many situations, the accreditation of the protocol and the face transplant programme is not enough to perform face transplantation. It is a requirement to have such accreditation. However, in most of the cases, RECs solicit to review every case with an indication for a face transplantation on an individual basis to make a case-by-case ethical deliberation and accreditation.

4.6 Appendix 4.1: The Helsinki Declaration

Adopted by the 18th WMA General Assembly, Helsinki, Finland, June 1964 and amended by the:

29th WMA General Assembly, Tokyo, Japan, October 1975

35th WMA General Assembly, Venice, Italy, October 1983

41st WMA General Assembly, Hong Kong, September 1989

48th WMA General Assembly, Somerset West, South Africa, October 1996

52nd WMA General Assembly, Edinburgh, Scotland, October 2000

53rd WMA General Assembly, Washington, DC, USA, October 2002

(Note of Clarification on paragraph 29 added)

55th WMA General Assembly, Tokyo, Japan, October 2004

(Note of Clarification on Paragraph 30 added)

59th WMA General Assembly, Seoul, Korea, October 2008

4.6.1 Introduction

1. The World Medical Association (WMA) has developed the Declaration of Helsinki as a statement of ethical principles for medical research involving human subjects, including research on identifiable human material and data. The Declaration is intended to be read as a whole, and each of its constituent paragraphs should not be applied without consideration of all other relevant paragraphs.

2. Although the Declaration is addressed primarily to physicians, the WMA encourages other participants in medical research involving human subjects to adopt these principles.

3. It is the duty of the physician to promote and safeguard the health of patients, including those who are involved in medical research. The physician's knowledge and conscience are dedicated to the fulfilment of this duty.

4. The Declaration of Geneva of the WMA binds the physician with the words "The health of my patient will be my first consideration," and the International Code of Medical Ethics declares that "A physician shall act in the patient's best interest when providing medical care".

5. Medical progress is based on research that ultimately must include studies involving human subjects. Populations that are underrepresented in medical research should be provided appropriate access to participation in research.

6. In medical research involving human subjects, the well-being of the individual research subject must take precedence over all other interests.

7. The primary purpose of medical research involving human subjects is to understand the causes, development and effects of diseases and improve preventive, diagnostic and therapeutic interventions (methods, procedures and treatments). Even the best current interventions must be evaluated continually through research for their safety, effectiveness, efficiency, accessibility and quality.

8. In medical practice and in medical research, most interventions involve risks and burdens.

9. Medical research is subject to ethical standards that promote respect for all human subjects and protect their health and rights. Some research populations are particularly vulnerable and need special protection. These include those who cannot give or refuse consent for themselves and those who may be vulnerable to coercion or undue influence.

10. Physicians should consider the ethical, legal and regulatory norms and standards for research involving human subjects in their own countries as well as applicable international norms and standards. No national or international ethical, legal or regulatory requirement should reduce or eliminate any of the protections for research subjects set forth in this Declaration.

4.6.2 Principles for All Medical Research

11. It is the duty of physicians who participate in medical research to protect the life, health, dignity, integrity, right to self-determination, privacy and confidentiality of personal information of research subjects.

12. Medical research involving human subjects must conform to generally accepted scientific principles and be based on a thorough knowledge of the scientific literature, other relevant sources of information and adequate laboratory and, as appropriate, animal experimentation. The welfare of animals used for research must be respected.

13. Appropriate caution must be exercised in the conduct of medical research that may harm the environment.

14. The design and performance of each research study involving human subjects must be clearly described in a research protocol. The protocol should contain a statement of the ethical considerations involved and should indicate how the principles in this Declaration have been addressed. The protocol should include information regarding funding, sponsors, institutional affiliations, other potential conflicts of interest, incentives for subjects and provisions for treating and/or compensating subjects who are harmed as a consequence of participation in the research study. The protocol should describe arrangements for post-study access by study subjects to interventions identified as beneficial in the study or access to other appropriate care or benefits.

15. The research protocol must be submitted for consideration, comment, guidance and approval to a research ethics committee before the study begins. This committee must be independent of the researcher, the sponsor and any other undue influence. It must take into consideration the laws and regulations of the country or countries in which the research is to be performed as well as applicable international norms and standards, but these must not be allowed to reduce or eliminate any of the protections for research subjects set forth in this Declaration. The committee must have the right to monitor ongoing studies. The researcher must provide monitoring information to the committee, especially information about any serious adverse events. No change to the protocol may be made without consideration and approval by the committee.

16. Medical research involving human subjects must be conducted only by individuals with the appropriate scientific training and qualifications. Research on patients or healthy volunteers requires the supervision of a competent and appropriately qualified physician or other health-care professional.

The responsibility for the protection of research subjects must always rest with the physician or other health-care professional and never the research subjects, even though they have given consent.

17. Medical research involving a disadvantaged or vulnerable population or community is only justified if the research is responsive to the health needs and priorities of this population or community and if there is a reasonable likelihood that this population or community stands to benefit from the results of the research.

18. Every medical research study involving human subjects must be preceded by careful assessment of predictable risks and burdens to the individuals and communities involved in the research in comparison with foreseeable benefits to them and to other individuals or communities affected by the condition under investigation.

19. Every clinical trial must be registered in a publicly accessible database before recruitment of the first subject.

20. Physicians may not participate in a research study involving human subjects unless they are confident that the risks involved have been adequately assessed and can be satisfactorily managed. Physicians must immediately stop a study when the risks are found to outweigh the potential benefits or when there is conclusive proof of positive and beneficial results.

21. Medical research involving human subjects may only be conducted if the importance of the objective outweighs the inherent risks and burdens to the research subjects.

22. Participation by competent individuals as subjects in medical research must be voluntary. Although it may be appropriate to consult family members or community leaders, no competent individual may be enrolled in a research study unless he or she freely agrees.

23. Every precaution must be taken to protect the privacy of research subjects and the confidentiality of their personal information and to minimise the impact of the study on their physical, mental and social integrity.

24. In medical research involving competent human subjects, each potential subject must be adequately informed of the aims, methods, sources of funding, any possible conflicts of interest, institutional affiliations of the researcher, the anticipated benefits and potential risks of the study and the discomfort it may entail and any other relevant aspects of the study. The potential subject must be informed of the right to refuse to participate in the study or to withdraw consent to participate at any time without reprisal. Special attention should be given to the specific information needs of individual potential subjects as well as to the methods used to deliver the information. After ensuring that the potential subject has understood the information, the physician or another appropriately qualified individual must then seek the potential subject's freely given informed consent, preferably in writing. If the consent cannot be expressed in writing, the non-written consent must be formally documented and witnessed.

25. For medical research using identifiable human material or data, physicians must normally seek consent for the collection, analysis, storage and/or reuse. There may be situations where consent would be impossible or impractical to obtain for such research or would pose a threat to the validity of the research. In such situations the research may be done only after consideration and approval of a research ethics committee.

26. When seeking informed consent for participation in a research study, the physician should be particularly cautious if the potential subject is in a dependent relationship with the physician or may consent under duress. In such situations the informed consent should be sought by an appropriately qualified individual who is completely independent of this relationship.

27. For a potential research subject who is incompetent, the physician must seek informed consent from the legally authorised representative. These individuals must not be included in a research study that has no likelihood of benefit for them unless it is intended

to promote the health of the population represented by the potential subject, the research cannot instead be performed with competent persons and the research entails only minimal risk and minimal burden.

28. When a potential research subject who is deemed incompetent is able to give assent to decisions about participation in research, the physician must seek that assent in addition to the consent of the legally authorised representative. The potential subject's dissent should be respected.

29. Research involving subjects who are physically or mentally incapable of giving consent, for example, unconscious patients, may be done only if the physical or mental condition that prevents giving informed consent is a necessary characteristic of the research population. In such circumstances the physician should seek informed consent from the legally authorised representative. If no such representative is available and if the research cannot be delayed, the study may proceed without informed consent provided that the specific reasons for involving subjects with a condition that renders them unable to give informed consent have been stated in the research protocol and the study has been approved by a research ethics committee. Consent to remain in the research should be obtained as soon as possible from the subject or a legally authorised representative.

30. Authors, editors and publishers all have ethical obligations with regard to the publication of the results of research. Authors have a duty to make publicly available the results of their research on human subjects and are accountable for the completeness and accuracy of their reports. They should adhere to accepted guidelines for ethical reporting. Negative and inconclusive as well as positive results should be published or otherwise made publicly available. Sources of funding, institutional affiliations and conflicts of interest should be declared in the publication. Reports of research not in accordance with the principles of this Declaration should not be accepted for publication.

4.6.3 Additional Principles for Medical Research Combined with Medical Care

31. The physician may combine medical research with medical care only to the extent that the research is justified by its potential preventive, diagnostic or therapeutic value and if the physician has good reason to believe that participation in the research study will not adversely affect the health of the patients who serve as research subjects.

32. The benefits, risks, burdens and effectiveness of a new intervention must be tested against those of the best current proven intervention, except in the following circumstances:
    - The use of placebo, or no treatment, is acceptable in studies where no current proven intervention exists.
    - Where for compelling and scientifically sound methodological reasons, the use of placebo is necessary to determine the efficacy or safety of an intervention, and the patients who receive placebo or no treatment will not be subject to any risk of serious or irreversible harm. Extreme care must be taken to avoid abuse of this option.

33. At the conclusion of the study, patients entered into the study are entitled to be informed about the outcome of the study and to share any benefits that result from it, for example, access to interventions identified as beneficial in the study or to other appropriate care or benefits.

34. The physician must fully inform the patient which aspects of the care are related to the research. The refusal of a patient to participate in a study or the patient's decision to withdraw from the study must never interfere with the patient–physician relationship.

35. In the treatment of a patient, where proven interventions do not exist or have been ineffective, the physician, after seeking expert advice, with informed consent from the patient or a legally authorised representative, may use an unproven intervention if in the physician's judgement it offers hope of saving

life, re-establishing health or alleviating suffering. Where possible, this intervention should be made the object of research, designed to evaluate its safety and efficacy. In all cases, new information should be recorded and, where appropriate, made publicly available.

4.7   Appendix 4.2: The Code of Nuremberg

1. The voluntary consent of the human subject is absolutely essential.

   This means that the person involved should have legal capacity to give consent; should be so situated as to be able to exercise free power of choice, without the intervention of any element of force, fraud, deceit, duress, over-reaching or other ulterior form of constraint or coercion; and should have sufficient knowledge and comprehension of the elements of the subject matter involved, as to enable him to make an understanding and enlightened decision. This latter element requires that, before the acceptance of an affirmative decision by the experimental subject, there should be made known to him the nature, duration and purpose of the experiment, the method and means by which it is to be conducted, all inconveniences and hazards reasonably to be expected and the effects upon his health or person, which may possibly come from his participation in the experiment.

   The duty and responsibility for ascertaining the quality of the consent rests upon each individual who initiates, directs or engages in the experiment. It is a personal duty and responsibility which may not be delegated to another with impunity.

2. The experiment should be such as to yield fruitful results for the good of society, unprocurable by other methods or means of study and not random and unnecessary in nature.

3. The experiment should be so designed and based on the results of animal experimentation and a knowledge of the natural history of the disease or other problem under study that the anticipated results will justify the performance of the experiment.

4. The experiment should be so conducted as to avoid all unnecessary physical and mental suffering and injury.

5. No experiment should be conducted where there is an a priori reason to believe that death or disabling injury will occur except, perhaps, in those experiments where the experimental physicians also serve as subjects.

6. The degree of risk to be taken should never exceed that determined by the humanitarian importance of the problem to be solved by the experiment.

7. Proper preparations should be made and adequate facilities provided to protect the experimental subject against even remote possibilities of injury, disability or death.

8. The experiment should be conducted only by scientifically qualified persons. The highest degree of skill and care should be required through all stages of the experiment of those who conduct or engage in the experiment.

9. During the course of the experiment, the human subject should be at liberty to bring the experiment to an end, if he has reached the physical or mental state, where continuation of the experiment seemed to him to be impossible.

10. During the course of the experiment, the scientist in charge must be prepared to terminate the experiment at any stage, if he has probable cause to believe, in the exercise of the good faith, superior skill and careful judgement required of him, that a continuation of the experiment is likely to result in injury, disability or death to the experimental subject.

Trials of War Criminals before the Nuremberg Military Tribunals under Control Council Law No. 10, vol. 2. Washington, D.C.: U.S. Government Printing Office; 1949. p. 181–2.

Functional Anatomy and Types of Face Transplants

5

Abstract

The bases of vascularised composite tissue allotransplantation rely on general principles of plastic and reconstructive surgery and on modern reconstructive microsurgery. In traditional autotransplantation, soft tissues in the form of flaps or vascularised anatomical parts are autotransplanted to another part of the same patient in order to reconstruct a defect caused by trauma, burns, atrophy or tumour ablation. Nonvascularised grafts survive by diffusion of nutrients until a new capillary network is created. In contrast, flaps do survive by a complete autonomous vascularisation created by microanastomosis between donor and recipient vessels. For years, these types of flaps have been used in reconstructive surgery, especially for head and neck reconstruction, breast reconstruction and lower limb salvage. An important clinical and experimental research has been implemented during the past two decades to provide evidence of the vascularisation of soft tissues and to develop new types of flaps to form and develop modern plastic reconstructive surgery.

The bases of vascularised composite tissue allotransplantation rely on general principles of plastic and reconstructive surgery and on modern reconstructive microsurgery. In traditional autotransplantation, soft tissues in the form of flaps or vascularised anatomical parts are autotransplanted to another part of the same patient in order to reconstruct a defect caused by trauma, burns, atrophy or tumour ablation. Nonvascularised grafts survive by diffusion of nutrients until a new capillary network is created. In contrast, flaps do survive by a complete autonomous vascularisation created by micro-anastomosis between donor and recipient vessels (Fig. 5.1). For years, these types of flaps have been used in reconstructive surgery, especially for head and neck reconstruction, breast reconstruction and lower limb salvage. An important clinical and experimental research has been implemented during the past two decades to provide evidence of the vascularisation of soft tissues (Table 5.1) and to develop new types of flaps (Figs. 5.2 and 5.3) to form and develop modern plastic reconstructive surgery.

Survival of microvascular flaps depends on an adequate inflow and outflow of vascularisation.

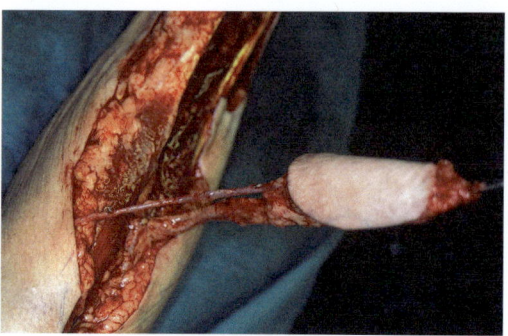

Fig. 5.1 Flaps are the basis of reconstructive microsurgery. Correct anastomosis between flap vessels and recipient's vessels (either termino-terminal or termino-lateral) is necessary for flap survival

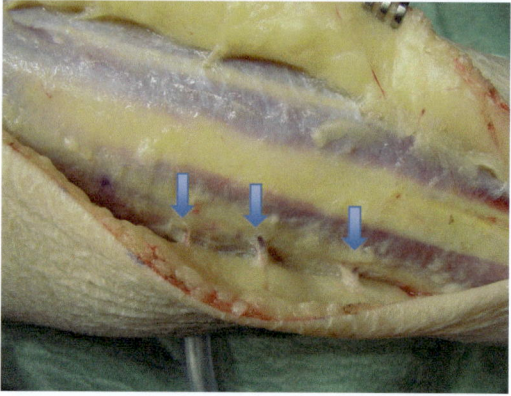

Fig. 5.2 Perforator vessels are the workhorse for new techniques (i.e. keystone flaps, freestyle flaps) and new reconstructive concepts. Arrows signal direct and musculocutaneous perforators

Table 5.1 Common flaps utilised in reconstructive surgery

1. Random local or regional flap (there is not any pedicle identified)
2. Axial pattern skin flaps (direct arteries to a cutaneous territory; i.e. groin flap)
3. Fasciocutaneous flaps (fascia, fat and skin, vascularisation through fascial feeders; i.e. radial forearm flap)
4. Perforator flaps (direct or indirect vessels that pierce fascia/muscle to vascularised soft tissues; i.e. deep inferior epigastric artery perforator [DIEAP] flap)
5. Muscle flaps (named muscle with its vascular(s) pedicle(s); may include nerve; i.e. latissimus dorsi muscle flap)
6. Musculocutaneous flaps (Muscle flaps with a skin and fat paddle vascularised through musculocutaneous feeders)
7. Osteocutaneous flaps (bone and skin ± muscle, through direct vessels and feeders; i.e. fibula flap)
8. Keystone flaps (locoregional flaps based on fascial/direct perforators/feeders)
9. Freestyle flaps (free or pedicle perforator flaps based on perforators of any given territory; identified by Doppler and designed ad hoc)
10. Various: free vascularised nerve flaps, bone flaps, composite flaps, chimera flaps, prefabricated flaps, etc.)

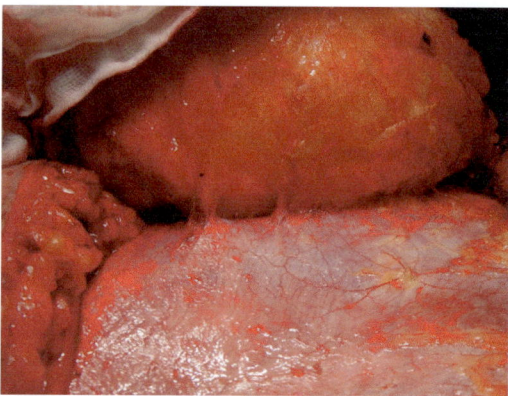

Fig. 5.3 Perforator vessels from the deep epigastric artery and vein form the vascular network for DIEAP flaps, commonly utilised in breast reconstruction

It is not only a question of a correct and efficient microvascular anastomosis and good recreation of an anatomical vascular network, but also of a sufficient and balanced blood flow through the entire transplanted tissues. Similarly, functional and sensory recovery relies on neurotisation of muscle units and excellency on neurorrhaphies between

donor and recipient nerves that allow scarless neural union that promotes ingrown of axons into the transplanted nerves (Fig. 5.4). The same general principles do apply to face allografts, which depend on a correct vascularisation and functional recovery from different vascular and neural anastomosis between the graft vessels and nerves and recipient vessels and nerves in the cervical and face areas of the recipient. The basis for a robust flap and efficient surgical technique resides on proficiency in reconstructive surgery and anatomic knowledge, often gained in the anatomy room and experimental microvascular lab.

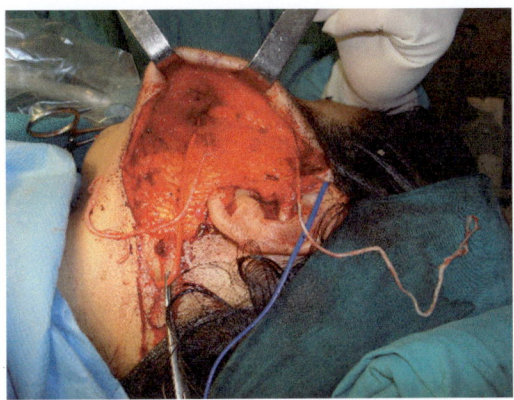

Fig. 5.4 Excellency in microsurgical technique is necessary to obtain good outcomes. Function depends on correct nerve coaptation, similarly to that obtained in face reanimation. Cross-face nerve grafts from sural nerves are anastomosed to face branches on the healthy hemiface and transposed to the contralateral side

5.1   Relevant Anatomy in Face Transplantation

Complete knowledge of anatomy of blood vessels and nerves and other anatomical units in the face and neck region is fundamental for the success of face transplantation. It is very important to understand the microvascular and macrovascular anatomy in order to include the specific vascularisation of any type of face VCA graft in the surgical approach.

5.1.1   Arterial Anatomy

The carotid artery axis is the main arterial network that forms the anatomical basis for face transplantation. Dissection of the common carotid artery is necessary for vascular cannulation in face transplants that receive the preservation fluid infusion in the absence of an intrathoracic approach. Face transplants that require a longer vascular axis for revascularisation require common carotid artery dissection in order to provide an extra length. The internal carotid artery and the vertebral artery do not play any role in face transplantation. They must be preserved, though, to avoid any cerebrovascular risk in the recipient.

They do have rich collateral anastomosis, especially the supraorbital artery, supratrochlear and the dorsal nasal artery. The external carotid artery and its terminal branches (in particular face, lingual and superficial temporal arteries) are the main branches for revascularisation and constitute the workhorses for face transplantation (Fig. 5.5).

The superior thyroid artery is the first branch of the external carotid. It does not play a significant role in face allograft procurement, although it is of interest in case it is necessary for revascularisation in the recipient, similarly to the approach utilised in head and neck reconstruction. The ascendant pharyngeal artery does not play any role in face transplantation either, since the posterior soft tissues receive sufficient vascularisation from collaterals in case the oropharynx is included in the transplant. The relevance of the lingual artery resides in its vascularisation of the tongue and related territories. It should be included in the dissection in case the tongue is included in the transplant. If it is necessary, it is advised to harvest in continuity with the external carotid artery and the face artery; in order to facilitate dissection, assure good blood supply to all territories and to perform an easy anastomosis end to end to the recipient's external carotid artery. The occipital artery is the following branch of the external carotid. It is seldom included in the allograft, and it should be considered when the whole scalp is to be transplanted. However, dissection is difficult and the alternative should constitute the superficial temporal artery.

The face artery is the workhorse vessel in face transplantation. Experimental and clinical experience provides the evidence that the entire face can be effectively vascularised by the face arteries. Good blood supply is observed in all territories. Therefore, including the superficial temporal vessels may not improve blood supply. It does, on the other hand, increase the complexity of the dissection, especially when a dissection in continuity with the external carotid and the face artery is contemplated. However, if a significant portion of the scalp is to be included in the transplant, it is necessary to include this

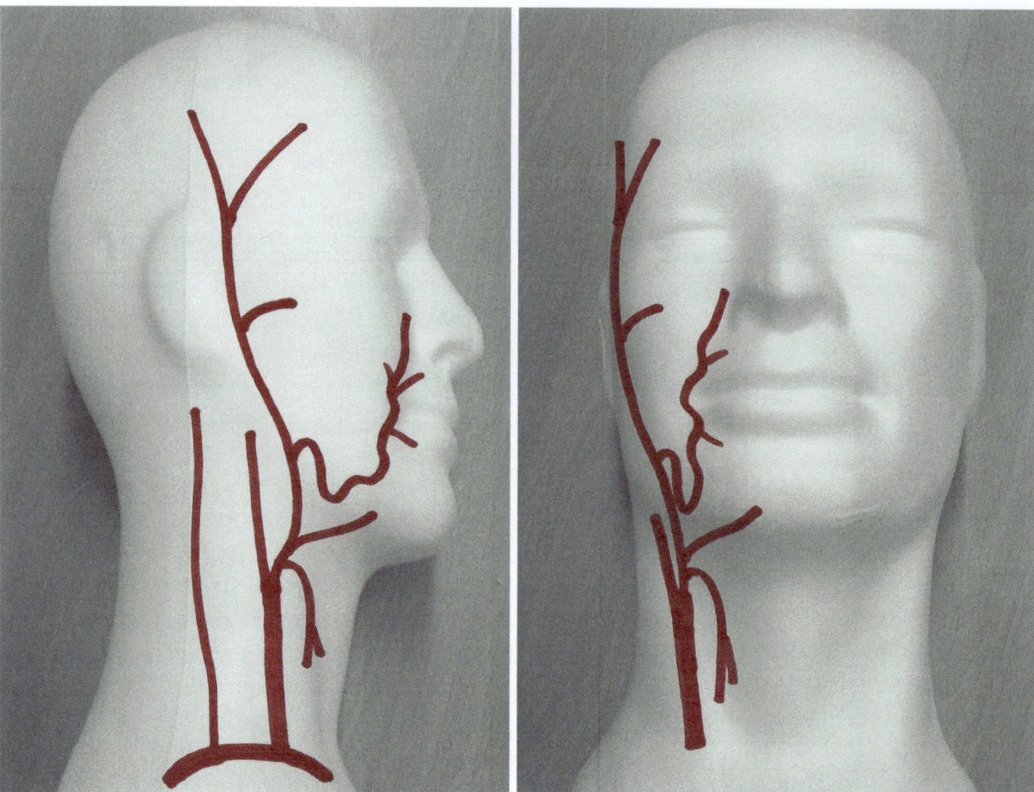

Fig. 5.5 Main arterial axis of the face and neck. Relevant arterial vessels for face VCA include face, temporal and external carotid artery

vessel either in a separate anastomosis or in an in-continuity dissection. The face artery follows a tortuous route in the upper portion of the neck, pierces the submandibular gland and emerges under the mandible before crossing this bone superficially. It networks in the face tissues providing different side branches (mentonian, labials), finishing in the lateral nasal artery, where it networks with branches of the internal carotid artery. In clinical cases, it has been observed a complete vascularisation of the entire face with pulsate bleeding on the contralateral face artery and in the posterior part of the soft tissues, including the face bone skeleton.

The internal maxillary artery is one of the major blood vessels in the mid-face. It does emerge posterior to the mandibular condyle and provides significant branches to the face, especially to the mandible and maxilla. Experimental and clinical evidence suggests that it may be ligated during face graft dissection. It does not

increase the risk for devascularisation, since face bones are well irrigated through the face artery.

The superficial temporal vessels constitute the end terminal branches of the external carotid artery. They may be included separately in the face graft or be included in a dissection in continuity with the external carotid artery, joining in this vascular plexus with the face artery. They contribute to the vascularisation of the forehead, scalp, ear and the lateral part of the face. However, unless a major part of the scalp and ears are necessary, they may be sacrificed, since sufficient blood supply is carried through the face artery axis.

5.1.2 Venous Anatomy

Correct and efficient outflow is necessary to provide a competent flap that does not show

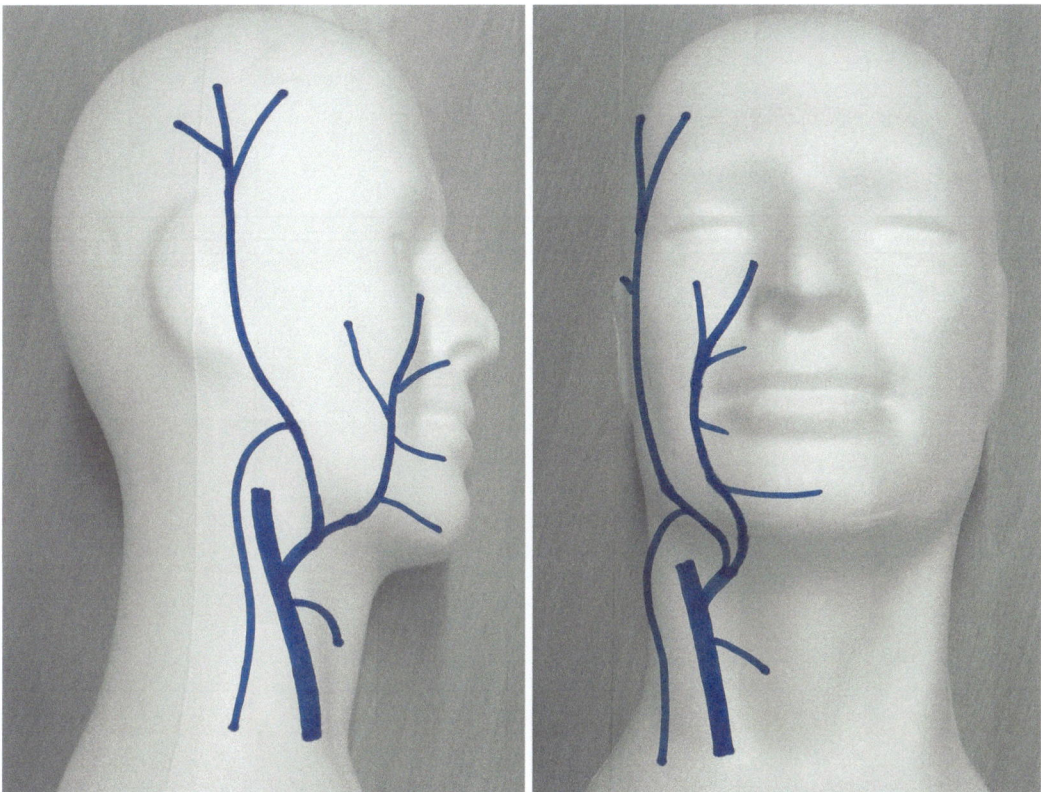

Fig. 5.6 Good venous return can be achieved with the inclusion of the face veins and external jugular vein. The retromandibular and internal jugular may be included in extensive VCA grafts

any signs of venous congestion and facilitates complete survival of the transplanted tissues. All major veins in the head and neck run parallel to the arterial axis. The only and extremely relevant exemption is the face vein (Fig. 5.6). The face vein has a much more posterior course than the face artery. Its course is linear (in comparison to the tortuous course of face artery). It receives many collateral branches and joins the superficial temporal vein just to form a main trunk before branching into the internal jugular vein. In face transplants that include the mandible, the retromandibular veins should also be included to increase the venous drainage of the transplant. The dissection may include part of the internal jugular to allow extra length in case it is necessary for the recipient's revascularisation. In case it is utilised, an end-to-side anastomosis is advised. Depending on the superficial venous architec-

ture and the type of transplant that has been designed, the external jugular vein may be included in the transplant to augment the venous drainage. A careful dissection must include all connections with the superficial network, superficial temporal vessels and face vein network. Depending on the complexity of the superficial venous drainage, excessive soft tissue dissection should be avoided to prevent face vessel damage.

In general terms, existing recipient's vessels, especially internal jugular veins, should suffice to allow for good face graft drainage. However, some cases, depending on the type of deformity, may present with a limited number of recipient veins for anastomosis. Under these circumstances, the cephalic vein may be freed and dissected and turned to an upward position to allow an extra venous anastomosis.

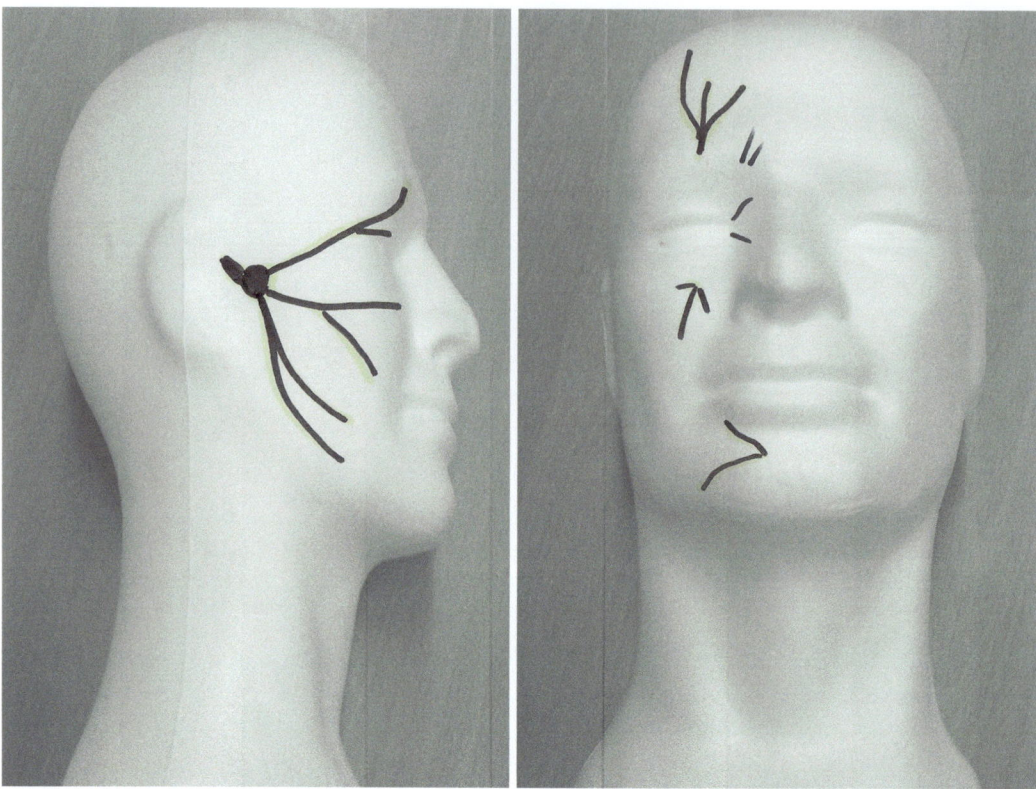

Fig. 5.7 Trigeminal branches should be included in every VCA face graft in order to obtain the best sensation and function. All three branches and lingual nerve are necessary in full face grafts and/or tongue

5.1.3 Nerve Anatomy

Vascular anatomy, proficiency in dissection and patent microvascular anastomosis are necessary for the success of face VCA. However, sensitive and motor nerves are extremely relevant and important to achieve the main objective of face transplantation: improvement of quality of life, overcome disability and reintegrate into society. In ideal circumstances, all nerves should be repaired. Nonetheless, in some patients (especially in trauma cases), nerves are severely damaged or absent. In such circumstances only those that can be identified may be repaired allowing enough recovery of function. The length of the nerves and their emergence through skull base foramens may limit some of the nerve repairs, thus nerve grafts might be necessary. Every attempt, though, should be made to perform a direct repair between nerve endings in order to

speed up recovery. However, when necessary, nerve grafts are utilised in order to allow a tension-free suture. From the motor functional standpoint, the most important cranial nerves are the face nerve and the motor branches of the trigeminal (mastication), whereas sensation and taste are controlled by sensitive trigeminal nerves. The hypoglossal nerves should also be included in the transplant should a tongue transplant be planned.

5.1.3.1 Trigeminal Nerve

The trigeminal nerve is the biggest cranial nerve, emerging from multiple skull base foramens (orbital fissure for the ophthalmic nerve (V1), round foramen for the maxillary nerve (V2) and the oval foramen for the mandibular nerve (V3)) (see Fig. 5.7). The ophthalmic nerve courses across the superior part of the orbit and emerges in the forehead through the supraorbital foramen (or fissure in some cases). It is responsible for the sensation of the forehead and most of the scalp. The maxillary nerve branches in multiple nerves, and it is responsible for the sensation of the central part of the face including the lower eyelid, the inferior part of the nose, upper lip, maxilla and gingival area. Even though it emerges through different maxillary foramens, the main branch of maxillary nerve is the infraorbital nerve, located below the orbit. This nerve should be considered in any face transplant in order to achieve the maximum sensory recovery in the mid- and lower face. The most inferior branch of the trigeminal nerve is the mandibular nerve. It provides sensation to areas of the tongue, the lower third of the face, lower gingival area and intraoral mucosa. The terminal branch of the mandibular nerve enters the mandible through the alveolar canal, turning into the inferior alveolar nerve. It emerges through the mental foramen to form the mentonian nerve, branching in the chin and lower lip. It should be included in the face transplant if a pure soft tissue transplant is considered. In turn, if the mandible is included, the nerve is either harvested on the skull base or above the entrance to the alveolar canal. When a tongue transplant is considered, the lingual nerve must be included in the graft, either in continuity with the mandibular nerve or as an individual nerve. Motor nerves include the masticator nerves for the masseter, temporal and pterygoids (harvested either as individual nerves or en bloc in type B transplants) and other muscles involved in deglutition and speech (mylohyoid, anterior belly of the digastric muscle, tensor veli palatini muscle and tensor tympani muscle).

5.1.3.2 Face Nerve

The cranial nerve VII (face) emerges through the stylomastoid foramen. Identification of face nerves during face graft procurement and transplantation does not differ from the dissection technique that is commonly used in traditional face nerve surgery. Dissection starts by identifying the main truck underneath the cartilaginous ear canal. It is advised to obtain the maximum length of face branches in order to ease the recipient's neurorrhaphy. Recipient's intact

branches are left intact, although it is imperative to obtain the most efficient function after face transplantation. It is not uncommon to sacrifice some branches and muscles in the recipient to provide undamaged nerves and muscles. The face nerve divides in the parotid in the main five face branches. The anatomy may vary: surgeons may encounter two main branches dividing in the final terminal nerves, although some anatomical variants may be present. Every effort must be executed to include all desired nerves and muscles in the transplant, since face function is a must in face transplantation to improve quality of life in face transplant recipients (Fig. 5.8).

Innervation of the Tongue: Complete sensory restoration of tongue function includes the lingual nerve (trigeminal branch (V3), provides sensation to the anterior two-thirds of the tongue), chorda tympani (provides taste sensation to the anterior two-thirds of the tongue) and glossopharyngeal nerve (cranial nerve IX, provides sensation and taste to the posterior one-third of the tongue). Motor function is provided by the hypoglossal nerve (easily identified in the superior part of the neck), which is responsible for most of the tongue movements. Even though it is very important to provide as much tongue function as possible, complete restoration of the tongue (especially taste and sensation) is limited by the posterior and deep location of all nerves and their short course in the skull base.

5.2   Types of Face Transplants

The classification of face transplants is, in general terms, straightforward. Depending on the quantity of tissue that is transplanted in any given transplant, face transplantation is classified as partial or total/full-face transplantation. It refers to classical or traditional reconstructive face surgery in which the reconstruction of face structures is termed either partial (parts of the anatomic unit are reconstructed) or total/full in which the whole anatomy is repaired. When the former is applied to face transplantation, the general classification stands as:

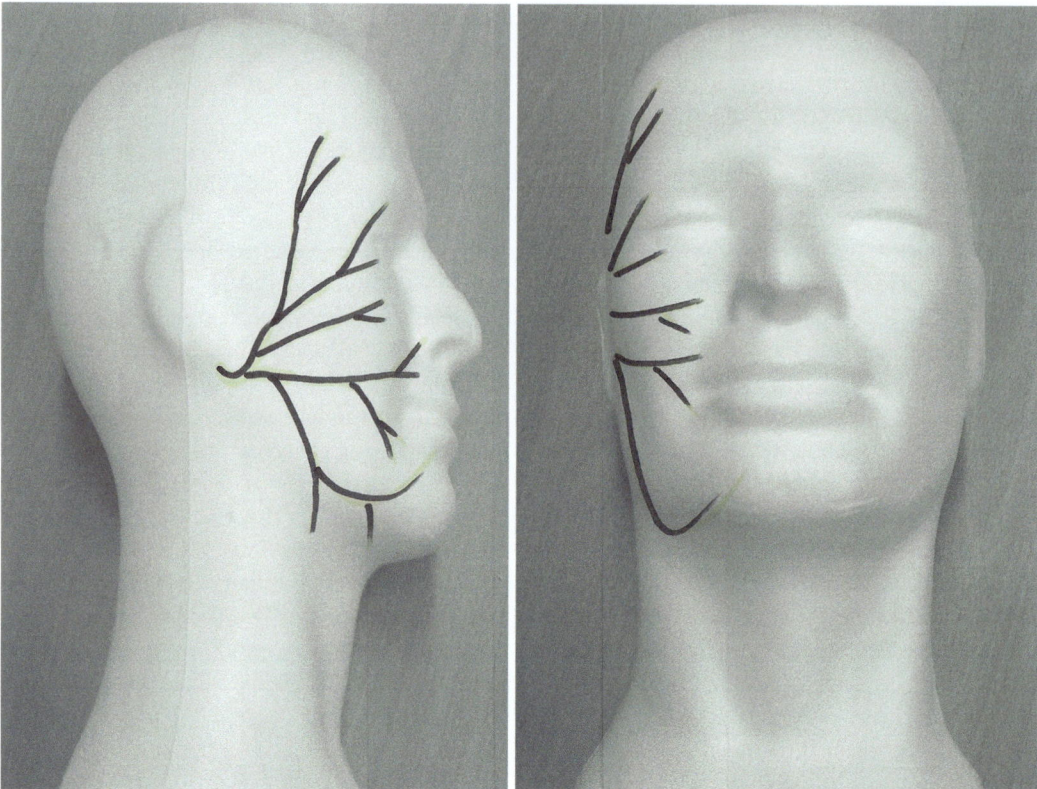

Fig. 5.8 Main branches of the face nerve. It is mandatory to include all motor nerve for correct functional outcome

- *Partial transplantation:* parts of the face are transplanted either as subunits or units. One or many face units are included in the transplant.
- *Total/full transplantation:* the whole face is transplanted as a graft, similarly to solid organ transplantation.

Dr. Lengele, though, has provided face VCA surgeons with a classification that combines the concepts of face anatomy and reconstructive surgery, making a more practical and useful classification that includes all types of face transplants.

Lengele's classification subdivides face transplantation into five types of face transplants, depending on the type of tissues and areas that are transplanted. It also takes into consideration the depth of the transplants and the inclusion of bones into the transplants. Each type of trans-

plant can be subdivided depending on whether the transplant includes face bones. Type A transplants include soft tissues only, whereas type B transplants include different amounts of face bones.

5.2.1 Type I Face Transplant (Lower Central)

This constitutes a face transplant that includes the inferior third of the face. It commonly includes the nose, lips and chin area (Fig. 5.9). In a type B, this type of transplant would include the mandible or parts of it. Zygomatic, buccal and mandibular branches of the face nerve reinnervate the muscles. The sensitive nerves of the allograft are the mental and infraorbital nerves. It is well vascularised by the face pedicles.

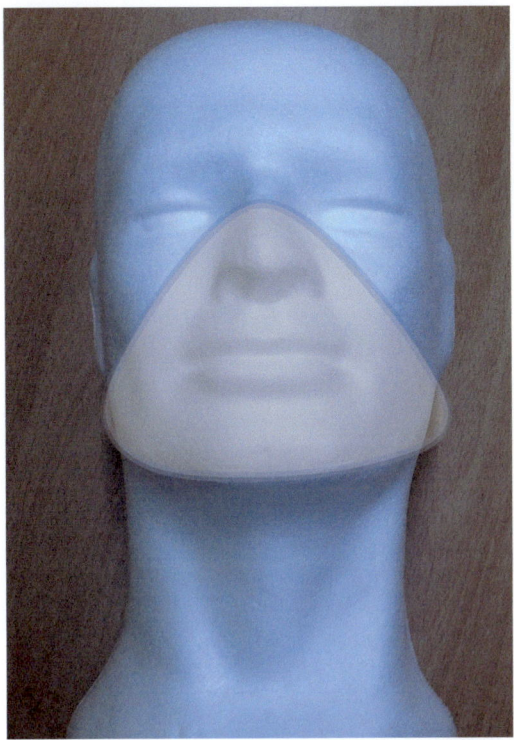 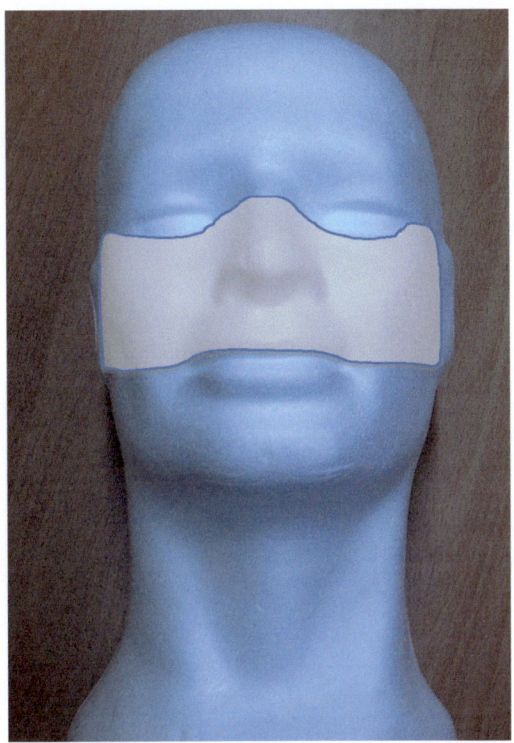

Fig. 5.9 Lower face VCA graft (type I). It commonly includes the chin, lips and nose. Vascularisation depends on both face arteries. Main motor branches include buccal, mandibular and zygomatic face nerves. The mental and infraorbital nerves provide sensation. Type B transplants may include the mandible and maxilla

Fig. 5.10 Mid-face VCA graft (type II). The cheeks, upper lip and nose are included in this type of transplant. It may be combined with type I. A combination of types I and II has been used in several face transplantation cases. Vascularisation depends mainly on face vessels. Main motor branches are the buccal and zygomatic branches, whereas sensation depends on the infraorbital nerve. Type B transplants may include zygomatic bones and maxilla

This was the world's first face transplantation ever, performed on November 2005 in Amiens, France (Dr. Devauchelle and team).

5.2.2 Type II Face Transplant (Mid Central)

The nose, upper lip, cheeks and mimic muscles are commonly transplanted in this type of VCA graft. It may include also the inferior part of the face, constituting then a true inferior face VCA graft (Fig. 5.10). The maxilla and parts of the mandible are bones included in a type II B face transplant. Vascularisation is obtained by the face pedicles, and it should include the infraorbital nerve and the zygomatic and buccal rami of the face nerve.

5.2.3 Type III Face Transplant (Upper Face)

This type of transplant includes the forehead, eyelids and root of the nose and mimic muscles (Fig. 5.11). Bone is not transplanted in this type of transplant. However, depending on the requirements of the recipient, parts of the nose and/or zygoma may be included. It is raised on the two temporal pedicles. The frontal and zygomatic

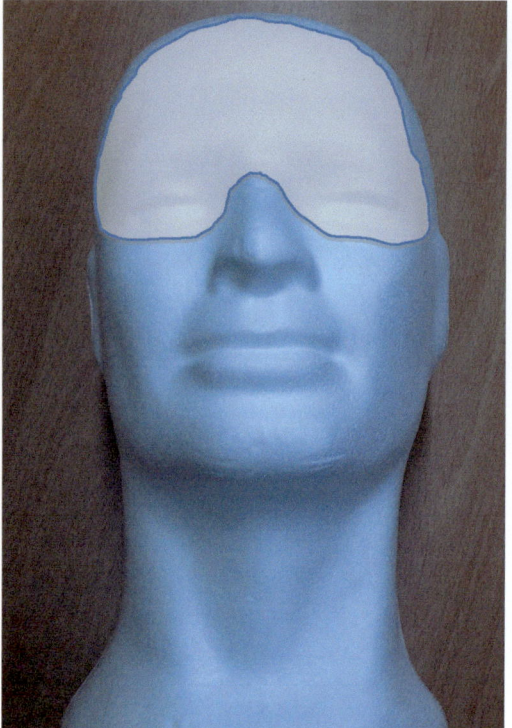

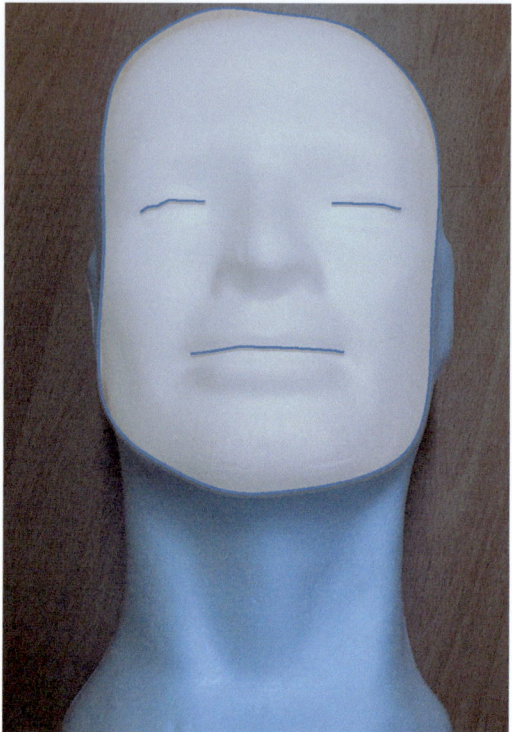

Fig. 5.11 Upper face VCA graft (type III). It includes the eyelids, temporal and forehead tissues. Motor branches depend on the orbicularis oculi and frontal nerves. Sensation is mainly through the supraorbital nerve. The temporal vessels provide vascularisation. Type B transplants may include root of the nose, or zygomas

Fig. 5.12 Full-face transplant (type V, either A or B). It is a combination of type I + II + III. Face and temporal vessels provide vascularisation. They may be dissected in continuity with the external carotid. It can include different amounts of intraoral tissues depending on the recipient's requirements

branches of the face nerve obtained restore muscle function.

5.2.4 Type IV Face Transplant

In this face transplant the skin and fat tissue of the face is transplanted. It constitutes a true resurfacing procedure of the entire face. This VCA graft is especially designed for burned patients. Although it has been termed full-face transplantation, it is indeed a partial allograft (type V allograft corresponds to a true full face transplant), restoring the surface of the face devoid of any muscle function. It does restore sensation, and all three trigeminal branches are included in the allograft. Vascularisation is obtained by face and temporal vessels harvested separately or in continuity with the external carotid artery

5.2.5 Type V Face Transplant (Full Face Transplant)

Type V transplants are full/total-face transplants (Fig. 5.12). They include all of the former (skin, fat, mimic muscles, nose, eyelids, lips, mucosa, etc.). Type B transplants would include the mandible, maxilla, zygomas and the nose. Recipient's requirements mandate which part of bony structures is transplanted. These are multisegments of composite transplants obtained on a single block of uniform thickness (types I, II and III). It contains all expression muscles, face motor branches and all three segmental branches of the trigeminal nerve, and it is vascularised by the face and temporal arches. The world's first full-face transplant was performed in Barcelona (Dr. Barret and team) in March 2010.

Evaluation of Candidates for Face Transplantation

6

Abstract

There has been an evolution in the management of face disfigurement in centres with face VCA programmes. Patients referred to plastic surgery clinics are no longer studied and offered traditional, though complex, reconstructive techniques. The deformity and the whole medical and psychological status of patients are taken into consideration, and all available options, including face transplantation, are considered in regard to expected aesthetic, anatomical and functional outcomes. This process allows plastic surgeons to estimate in whole the defect, deformity, functional and social impact and make a valid indication of the technique of choice for any given defect. Most of the patients will be offered and be reconstructed with classical reconstructive techniques, while only a few patients will enter the face transplant programme. In our hands, only 10–20 % of patients entering the face transplantation programme will end up with an indication and final ethical committee accreditation.

Patient selection in face transplantation is a complex process that starts with the indication for face transplantation, inclusive all psychological, ethical and legal issues, followed by a complete medical workup.

The evaluation of patients begins in the initial visit. The patient should be evaluated within a multidisciplinary team to make a full medical and biographical picture of the physical, functional, social and psychological deformity and disability and make a final indication for face vascularised composite tissue allotransplantation. In general terms, the technique, operation and some issues of transplant surgery are very similar to that encountered in other solid organ transplantation. However, when we consider in full patient evaluation and selection, there are significant differences that have to be taken into account.

There has been an evolution in the management of face disfigurement in centres with face VCA programmes. Patients referred to plastic surgery clinics are no longer studied and offered traditional, though complex, reconstructive techniques. The deformity and the whole medical and psychological status of patients are taken into consideration, and all available options, including face transplantation, are considered in regard to expected aesthetic, anatomical and functional outcomes. This process allows plastic surgeons to estimate in whole the defect, deformity, functional

J.P. Barret, V. Tomasello, *Face Transplantation: Principles, Techniques and Artistry*,
DOI 10.1007/978-3-662-45444-2_6, © Springer-Verlag Berlin Heidelberg 2015

and social impact and make a valid indication of the technique of choice for any given defect. Most of the patients will be offered and be reconstructed with classical reconstructive techniques, while only a few patients will enter the face transplant programme. In our hands, only 10–20 % of patients entering the face transplantation program will end up with an indication and final ethical committee accreditation.

6.1 The Initial Visit

Large tertiary institutions that have a long tradition in transplantation medicine and run a robust programme in plastic and reconstructive surgery normally host face transplantation programmes. Level I trauma centres, burn units or centres and superregional craniomaxillofacial programmes are usually normal referral units in such institutions.

The initial referral visit for face transplantation should not differ much to that usually in place for face reconstructive surgery. In practice, it is recommended that all patients be referred to the face reconstructive outpatient clinic for a complete initial visit where he/she may meet all surgical team members and a complete analysis of the problem be made. The rationale behind this approach resides on the basis that face transplantation is not a plain composite tissue allotransplantation venture but a complex reconstructive option, in which the reconstruction is performed by means of the allotransplantation of face units/anatomy and function. Evaluation of patients with severe face deformities then follow a step-wise manner in which all reconstructive options are taken into account and a final master plan for any given patient is delineated. It may include different classical techniques that may render a good final outcome of a definitive indication for face transplantation.

There exist few initial steps that need to be explored and fulfilled in order to plan a comprehensive evaluation for a face transplantation. During the initial visit, team members check all the inclusion and exclusion criteria for face transplantation; explore and analyse the patient's deformity, possible plastic surgery indications and

required techniques; and list all patient's complaints, aesthetic, functional deficits and patient's expectations (Fig. 6.1). During this initial visit, a complete blood test is run in order to rule out any formal contraindication for face transplantation. During this initial(s) visit(s) (it may be necessary to have different interviews with the patient), the patient is provided with all necessary information. It is mandatory that the patient receives all information regarding the positive, negative aspects of the procedure, risks and benefits and that he/she understand the experimental aspect of vascularised composite tissue allotransplantation. An introduction to the multidisciplinary team is also enforced and the requirement of different interviews with the core members of different specialists that will be required. Patients are also informed of the whole selection process and the administrative steps that must be followed:

- Full medical and surgical examination with any diagnostic laboratory, functional and radiologic examinations
- Psychological and psychiatric evaluation
- Psychosocial evaluation by social workers
- Informed consent for clinical experimental treatment
- Ethics committee submission if an indication for face transplantation is reached
- Submission to the health authorities (local and national transplantation bodies, organ procurement organizations)
- Final accreditation and search for donors

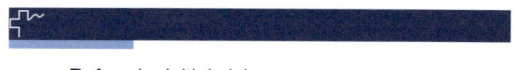

- Referral – initial visit
- Information + preliminary screening
- Indication for face Tx

- Hospital admission 2–3 weeks
- Full battery of tests

Fig. 6.1 Recommended process for the evaluation of face transplant recipients. Hospital admission allows for an effective process with good interaction with team members

Patients that are considered candidates for face transplantation are then admitted to the hospital. They are informed and warned that a hospital admission for a 2–3-week period may be necessary to fulfil all the tests and requirements according to the VCA face protocol. We have found that admitting patients to the plastic surgery ward is very valuable for both performing all necessary examinations and interviews in a timely fashion and for a good interaction of patients and their families with the transplantation team and ward nurses. During all long "stand-by" hours between tests and interviews, patient behaviour, social interaction, resilience and stress response can be evaluated. The report of caring nurses is extremely valuable to make a general picture of the psychosocial status of the patients and his/her social environment. Strong and weak points may be detected and encouraged or treated accordingly.

6.2 The Evaluation Process

It cannot be overstated that the initial(s) visit(s) is a key element of the evaluation process. During these visits the surgeon-in-chief and team members evaluate the face deformity and obtain a clear picture of the anatomic deformity, the functional impact and the general psychosocial status of the patients. Full information of the goals of face transplantation, benefits, risks and possible side effects, including death, are discussed. Patients reaching the evaluation process have understood and accepted the overall principles and goals of face transplantation, accepting a full examination with its possible positive or negative outcomes.

Different specialists, units and services are involved during the evaluation process. It is a thorough medical and surgical workup; hence, a case manager and a surgeon-in-chief that control the process and lead the process must pilot it. Plastic surgery specialists evaluate all questions and issues regarding the surgical aspect of the deformity (anatomic areas to be extirpated and donor tissue requirements). The former includes a full anthropomorphic evaluation,

physical examination (including radiologic evaluation) and skin phototype. Medical specialists of the face transplant team should evaluate the health status and well-being, paying a special attention to those conditions that currently contraindicate a vascularised composite tissue allotransplantation (malignant neoplasm, renal failure, hepatic insufficiency, ASA III or IV classification, etc.) and other medical conditions that merit attention in order to improve or treat them before the transplant. Some of these conditions may exacerbate with immunosuppression or contraindicate certain drug regimens. Psychologists and psychiatrists transplant specialists evaluate all patients. Special attention is focused to pre-existing pathology, normal or superior intelligence coefficient, previous adhesion to medications and medical treatments, etc. The psychological–psychiatric evaluation is then directed to develop a patient's profile, with an emphasis on the risk of abandon for immunosuppression, family and social support, pre- and posttransplant education, and produce an analysis and recommendations. A negative report from the transplant psychologist and psychiatrist contraindicates a face transplantation and is a formal exclusion criterion.

6.2.1 General Evaluation

The general evaluation of a patient being considered for a face transplantation does not differ much from other face plastic surgery patients. A general master plan has to be created; hence, information regarding medical status and anatomic and functional deformity should be gathered.

The patient has to be identified and all demographics recorded. Surgeons bear in mind that they may be entering a clinical research protocol and a special identifying number shall be assigned. Patient's telephone and relatives' telephone numbers are recorded for future direct contact. The disease (if any) and type of deformity are recorded and studied thoroughly. Height, weight and all anthropomorphic measurements are recorded (Table 6.1); a hand-held Doppler is

Table 6.1 Common anthropomorphic clinical measurements in face transplantation

1. Interpupillary distance
2. Intercanthal (external and internal) distance
3. Head perimeter (brow level)
4. Hairline–nasion distance
5. Nasal length
6. Upper lip–chin distance
7. Hairline–chin distance
8. Inter-preauricular distance

Table 6.2 Face general evaluation

1. Areas affected
2. Involvement of face sphincters (oral and orbital)
3. Cranial nerve involvement
4. Ocular status
5. Hearing status
6. Intraoral structures status

performed to assess the patency of face vessels and all results recorded.

A full history is next. Special attention is paid to allergies, medications and history of past surgeries and type, transfusion requirements and any history of transfusion reactions and any relevant past medical history. Immunosuppression drug protocols may produce different side effects; thus the medical history should focus on renal diseases, hepatic problems, cardiovascular and any other endocrine disturbances. Systemic hypertension, posttransplant diabetes, renal failure or hepatic insufficiency may develop after the transplant; consequently, any minor problems should be treated and resolved before the transplant. Important medical problems may contraindicate the face transplant. The type of nutrition and dietetic problems or deficiencies are recorded and type of airway assessed. It is not uncommon, especially in posttraumatic deformities that the patients present with a gastrostomy tube feeding and a patent tracheotomy. During the initial visit and the posterior general evaluation (together with the nutritional and anaesthetic assessment), the need for a gastrostomy tube feeding and a temporal tracheotomy is discussed with the patient if they are not yet in place. They may be necessary and ease the postoperative period.

The face examination is an important part of the general evaluation of the patient and will aid in the decision process for the formal indication and the type of transplant (Table 6.2). The type of deformity and aetiology is recorded. Areas affected are studied and evaluated. Any relevant defects, missing anatomy and altered function are recorded to make a general picture of the deformity and the functional and emotional impact of

the face disfigurement. Functional impact is best evaluated by the assessment of the visual, auditory and sensory and motor nerve status, together with an exploration and evaluation of the intraoral structures:

6.2.1.1 Cranial Nerve Status

Special attention should be paid to the ocular cranial nerves (cranial nerves III, IV and VI) in regard to eye movement and visual impairment; evaluation of the motor and sensitive branches of the trigeminal nerve (V), its function and the anatomical situation of the nerve must be explored; during face transplantation the first, second and third divisions are to be anastomosed to obtain excellent sensory outcomes. Face transplantation is a quality of life transplant, and faces transplanted must be sensitive, not merely functioning like a mask. The face nerve merits also a special word. The status of all face muscles and the function of the different branches and their anatomical status are also crucial for an optimal functional outcome. Cranial nerves IX, XI and XII are also assessed; special care must be paid when a face transplant that includes intraoral structures (soft palate, oropharynx, floor of the mouth and/or tongue) is considered.

6.2.1.2 Visual Status

There has been great debate so as to whether a face transplant is ever indicated in a blinded patient. Similarly to what occurred with the ethical, scientific and social process of face transplantation, the initial arguments against face transplantation in blinded patients have been answered by clinical practice. Excellent functional and psychological outcomes have been achieved in blinded patients. Quality of life has improved significantly in this group of patients, which signals that face transplantation is not merely an improvement in face appearance.

6.2.1.3 Hearing Impairment

Audition and external, middle and internal ear function and anatomy are assessed in a similar fashion. Hearing impairment is not a contraindication for face transplantation. It is important, though, to have a good and fluent communication with patients. Any hearing loss should be assessed and addressed, making any efforts for improvement. The status of the external ear is also examined. If a partial or total destruction of the external ear or auditory canal is present, they should be included in the specimen to be transplanted.

6.2.1.4 Intraoral Structures

Functional status of the intraoral structures, including speech, feeding and swallowing, is explored. Any deficits are noted, together with the status of the lip sphincter, palate, teeth, tongue, oropharynx and floor of the mouth. Any absent or destroyed anatomy must be delineated and included in the projected transplant specimen if deemed indicated. The external sphincter may be commonly involved in the deformity in most cases (it is a formal indication for face transplantation), whereas the internal structures are most often involved in tumours, postoncological deformities and gunshot injuries. Cranial nerves must be explored and any expected difficulties in neurotisation and reinnervation noted. Rehabilitation and speech pathology services must be consulted in order to complete the preoperative evaluation and determine the postoperative requirements. The exploration is completed with EMG exploration and imaging.

6.2.2 Laboratory Tests

Face transplantation is commonly being indicated for healthy individuals. The technique is in its initial phase, and patients that present with significant co-morbidities are excluded. During the general evaluation process, some system disturbances or concomitant diseases may be encountered. Patients are normally referred to team members for assessment. All altered tests and system alterations are treated and corrected prior to the surgical intervention. Those that cannot be corrected and may be exacerbated by immunosuppression are considered a contraindication unless the transplant is being indicated for a deformity that poses a higher risk than the disease. This situation is very rare and should be evaluated in depth by the team and be referred to the clinical ethics committee for counselling and deliberation.

Laboratory examination follows similar guidelines to those of solid organ transplantation. It must be noted, though, that patients may have received multiple transfusions (multiple operations, burns, etc.) and/or skin allografts (burns). Therefore, patients may have developed a positive cross-match or antibodies against tissues and HLA antigens.

A general analytical workup is performed (Table 6.3). It includes haematology (red blood cells, leucocytes, platelets and coagulation

Table 6.3 General laboratory tests

Haematology:
Haemoglobin, haematocrit, reticulocytes, platelet count, red blood cell physiology, leucocytes (with subtypes), coagulation study (prothrombin time, activated partial thromboplastin time [aPTT], thrombin time and fibrinogen)
Blood group and rhesus
Coombs tests
Hypercoagulation status study (if personal or family history)
Biochemistry:
Ions (sodium, potassium, chloride, CO_2, magnesium, zinc)
Calcium phosphate metabolism
Bilirubin (total and direct)
Alanine aminotransferase (ALT), aspartate aminotransferase (AST), gamma-glutamyl transpeptidase (GGT), alkaline phosphatase
Total proteins/albumin
Lipids
Total cholesterol
High-density lipoprotein (HDL) cholesterol
Low-density lipoprotein (LDL) cholesterol
Very low-density lipoprotein (VLDL) cholesterol
Triglycerides
Creatinine clearance

Table 6.4 Immunological laboratory studies

Tissue typing (HLA antigens)
Cross-match, PRA%
Immunoglobulins (A, M, G)
Lymphocyte subtype populations
Autoimmunity study

Table 6.5 Microbiology tests

Serology:
Cytomegalovirus (CMV)
Epstein–Barr virus (EBV)
Hepatitis A, B, C
HIV
Herpes simplex 1, 2, 6
Varicella zoster
Rubella
Parotiditis
Treponema pallidum (syphilis)
Tuberculosis (purified protein derivative [PPD])
Nasal Swab (methicillin-resistant *Staphylococcus aureus* [MRSA])
Tracheotomy swab/tracheal aspirate
Immigrants/endemic areas:
Regional mycosis
Malaria
Chagas disease
Strongyloidiasis

assay), a special coagulation panel study if a personal or family history of coagulation problems is encountered, and clinical biochemistry, including ions, calcium phosphate metabolisms, liver metabolism, lipids and creatinine clearance.

Another important part of the analytical study includes the immunological (Table 6.4) and infectious diseases studies (Table 6.5). Blood group and rhesus, tissue type, HLA antigens, immunoglobulins and lymphocyte subtypes are studied. As mentioned before, a detection panel for HLA antigen antibodies and an autoimmunity study are included. Correct outcomes in composite tissue allotransplantation depend on many variables, one of which is maintenance of healthy status with low risk of infections and as low as possible number of infectious episodes. During this phase of the evaluation, the infectious specialists explore serology status and past viral and bacterial infections. An important part

is viral infections, in special cytomegalovirus, Epstein–Barr, hepatitis panel, herpes and varicella zoster, syphilis, tuberculosis, nasal swab for MRSA and tracheotomy if applicable. Cytomegalovirus and Epstein–Barr viral infections are very relevant. CMV-negative patients should be protected for primary infection. Special attention should be paid to negative recipients of positive CMV donors. Some centres do not accept them as donors, being a contraindication for a face transplant under their protocol guidelines. We currently accept them and have not had any increased difficulty in the postoperative period. Positive Epstein–Barr needs to be monitored closely for malignant development. Other important issues are hepatitis C (some centres do not accept them as recipients) and human immunodeficiency virus (HIV) (not a contraindication). Centres considering patients from endemic areas for certain diseases or immigrants should run a panel for regional mycosis, malaria, Chagas' disease and strongyloidiasis. The transplant infectious disease specialist evaluates the patient and patient's results and any recommendations passed onto the rest of the team and the surgeon-in-chief. The immunology/infectious disease team is completed by preventive medicine. A specialist should be involved in the VCA team and be in close relationship with surgeons and transplant immunologists. Following the evaluation by surgeons and infectious disease specialists and the performance of the microbiology tests analysis, any relevant vaccines are administered to the patients to start with the prevention program. Main areas of intervention are hepatitis A and B, varicella zoster, rubella, parotiditis and current flu vaccination (in consideration to the different season's antigens).

6.2.3   Imaging and Other Special Explorations

A general preoperative workup is mandatory (Table 6.6). It includes the usual thorax X-ray examination, electrocardiogram and mammography if necessary. Other common X-ray examinations include orthopantomography and

Table 6.6 Imaging and other special explorations

1. Complete preoperative workup
   Thorax X-ray
   Electrocardiogram
   Mammography
   Orthopantomography and cephalometry
2. Face CT scan
3. Face MRI
4. Face angio-CT scan
5. EMG
6. Swallowing videoscope
7. Triple nasopharynx–larynx endoscopy
8. Upper and lower digestive tract endoscopy
9. Urological/gynaecological examination
10. PET scan, lung CT scan
11. Isotopic kidney scan

cephalometry, similarly to other craniomaxillo-face assessments.

The imaging exploration must be completed with a CT scan and magnetic resonance. These explorations aid in the assessment of the deformity, extension of the tumours if applicable and preparation for the surgical panning. The X-ray examination should be completed with an angio-CT scan (Fig. 6.2). This exploration provides relevant information regarding the vascular anatomy of the face structures, and it is very helpful in the preoperative planning. It allows for a full knowledge of the existing anatomy and an excellent preparation of the surgical plan, especially in

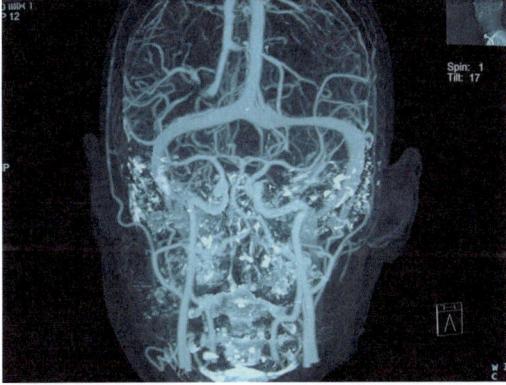

Fig. 6.2 Angio-CT Scan is highly recommended in the preoperative evaluation of face transplant recipients. Full knowledge of the existing anatomy and the vascular network is a must for a successful face transplantation procedure

regard to revascularisation. Many patients have been operated on in the past and face anatomy may be distorted. Some of these operations may include free microsurgical tissue transfers; hence, some of the regional arteries may not be available. The preoperative knowledge of all these issues allows for a complete planning and consideration of all techniques that will be necessary to perform a successful face transplantation (i.e. vein grafts, osteotomies, bone grafts, etc.).

Other explorations that are necessary to finalise the evaluation of the candidate include the evaluation of the functional status of some of the most relevant structures of face anatomy. They include electromyogram, with complete exploration of the function of face muscle and face branches, trigeminal branches and any necessary nerve conduction studies and nerve sensory potentials. Swallowing videoscope measures and explores the oropharynx and tongue function, together with a triple nasoendoscopy to assess the status of the nose, pharynx and larynx. It is also advised to perform a functional MRI to depict the functional cortical representation for scientific and clinical follow-up.

Digestive endoscopy (oesophagogastroduodenoscopy and colonoscopy) and urological examination and prostate cancer markers are indicated in patients with a personal or family history of malignant or premalignant neoplasms or in those patients over 50 years old. The complete workup detects any oncological potential in patients considered for VCA transplantation and allows for treatment or counselling if indicated. Patients with postoncological face deformities should follow similar workup, with completion of a PET scan to rule out any hidden malignancies. Smokers should be asked to stop the nicotine abuse, and both smokers and ex-smokers should follow a complete lung examination with lung functional analysis and thorax CT scan. Patients with an impaired or borderline renal function undergo an isotopic functional kidney scan and formal consultation with nephrology services.

The evaluation of the candidate is completed with consultation to relevant team specialists that shall be involved in the operative and postoperative planning and follow-up. Psychosocial specialists perform the most relevant part of the evaluation. Psychiatrist and psychologists evaluate the patient and perform all necessary tests and interviews to assess the indication for a face transplant. It has been mentioned before that a negative report from the psychological evaluation is a formal contraindication for VCA. Social services are similarly consulted for a complete social intervention, which assess not only the patient but also the family, home situation and social support. Any items for intervention are noted and explored. Other specialists that are involved in the evaluation at this stage are anaesthesiology (a formal preoperative examination and preparation for the procedure is depicted), preventive medicine (vaccinations and other general interventions, they liaise with social workers for the general domestic and social situation), infectious diseases, rehabilitation, nutrition (special attention is paid to the current nutritional status and the expected problems or issues to be encountered in the postoperative period, with special focus to the necessity for percutaneous gastrostomy enteral nutrition) and nephrology.

After completion of all formal clinical, laboratory, functional and imaging tests and explorations, a complete case report form is developed. All candidates that present no formal contraindications for face transplantation are informed of the outcome of the evaluation and receive an indication for a face transplantation. Patients are informed and all results discussed with them, with a special focus on the potential and individualised risks for the procedure. The proposed operative planning and the specific details of the operation are delineated, and the relevant issues regarding tissue donation, organ procurement, waiting lists and the overall process of solid organ and VCA transplantation are discussed in full. Special attention is paid to the experimental nature of VCA and possible outcomes, including death. Patients need to understand all these issues and understand in full the implications of face transplantation, the risks and the expected benefits. Patients that are well informed; understand the risks and benefits, outcomes and the transplantation process and have no contraindication for VCA are then con-

sidered formal candidates, and the treatment is offered. Informed consent follows.

The process is finalised with submission of the case report form, the informed consent and the psychological–psychiatric evaluation for consideration to the Ethics Committee. Ethics Committee submission is a consultation body, which delivers their consideration with positive or negative outcomes. Committees do not approve or disapprove treatments; they issue recommendations in any individual medical case concerning clinical practice. However, a negative outcome that cannot be corrected with revision of the indication and resubmission is considered a contraindication for VCA. A positive report from the Ethics Committee allows for final formal submission to the regional or national transplantation bodies for accreditation and organ procurement organizations for the search for donors.

6.3   Appendix 6.1: Informed Consent for Face Transplant Recipients

Patient Name:
  Passport Number/National ID Number:
  Hospital Number:
  Date of Birth:
  Diagnosis:
  Type of Proposed Transplantation:
1. What is a face transplantation?
    Face transplantation is an operation that is performed under general anaesthesia. During the intervention, through different incisions on the face, all deformed structures are removed and all necessary parts of the face from a cadaveric donor are implanted. The transplant may be total or only some parts of the face may be removed and implanted. The implant consists in the fixation with stitches and other surgical fixations to the face and the anastomosis (putting structures together) of vessels and nerves. If bones of the face are also transplanted, they are fixated with mini-plates and screws. Some persons may need vein or nerve grafts for the intervention (pieces of vessels and nerves from the same person or

from the cadaveric donor). If you do not have in place at the moment of the operation a tracheotomy (a hole on the throat to allow for breathing), this may be necessary if your surgeon or anaesthetist thinks so. The tracheotomy is normally closed few days after the operation when you can safely breathe on your own through the nose and mouth.

There exist different types of face transplants:

- Partial face transplantation (only part of the face is transplanted)
- Full/total face transplantation (the whole face is transplanted)

Depending on the type of structures that are deformed, there are also other types of transplants:

- Transplantation of skin and subcutaneous tissues
- Transplantation of skin, subcutaneous tissues and muscles
- Transplantation of skin, subcutaneous tissues, muscles and bone
- Transplantation of the tongue and intraoral structures
- All of the above

Your surgeon will inform you of the type of structures that need to be removed and transplanted.

Face transplantation is still a clinical experimental treatment, with long-term consequences and risks that are unknown. Consequently, the Ethics Committee and the Competent Legal Transplantation Bodies release authorisation on an individual basis.

2. Preoperative considerations

A multidisciplinary team evaluates patients, and different tests and explorations are performed. Following this evaluation, patients that fulfil all the requirements dictated by the approved protocol are considered candidates for a face transplantation. The former means that after full consideration of the risks and benefits of the proposed treatment, face transplantation is deemed the best alternative for the reconstruction of the face. The expected functional and anatomical reconstruction with traditional techniques cannot

achieve the projected outcome of a face transplantation.

When a donor is available, the recipient is selected according to his/her date of inclusion in the waiting list. This is made in full consideration of the biological and anatomical compatibility between the donor and the recipient.

The recipient that has been selected for face transplantation is then admitted to the hospital in order to update the preoperative check.

At this stage two situations may be encountered:

1. Following full evaluation of the donor and the recipient, donor is not considered a good match (it may be considered for another candidate). Under this circumstance the recipient is discharged and will reassume the search for donor (waiting list).
2. The donor is a good match and the transplant is carried out.
3. The operation

   Mean duration of surgeries varies; they may last between 15 and 24 h; some cases may require longer operative time. The operation consists in the substitution of all absent or deformed tissues and face structures by those obtained from a cadaveric donor. In order to obtain and restore the anatomy and function, it is necessary to perform microanastomosis of vessels and nerves and to adapt and fixate all transplanted structures

4. Survival

   Survival depends on different factors, some from donors and other from recipients: previous surgeries, vessel damage, complications, etc. Face transplantation is an extremely complex intervention that carries with a long operative time, large amount of blood transfusion and admission to the intensive care unit. Any procedures during this process have a significant risk: these are life-threatening situations and the possibility of death.

5. The postoperative period. What occurs after the transplant?

Right after the completion of the face transplantation, the patient will be admitted to the intensive care unit where you will be cared for by intensivists, surgeons, infectologists and the rest of the transplant team. You will be intubated and will receive the support of a ventilator (a special machine that will aid the respiration). For the first hours/days, you will be sedated with full intensive support. Your doctors will wake you up when they consider that there is no risk for your life. The time you will spend in the intensive care unit varies depending on the type of the transplant, your individual conditions and possible complications. When your doctors consider your status stable and risk free, you will be transferred to the plastic surgery ward where you will stay until the moment you are discharged home. You should expect a long stay in the hospital, normally dictated by the recovery and the stability of tests and your ability to cope with daily living activities.

Following discharge, you will be asked to attend our clinic on a regular basis. Hospital admissions for immunological, infectious or side effect complications are not uncommon. You will receive immunosuppressive drugs for the rest of your life in order to prevent the rejection of the transplant. If you stop taking these medications, you will suffer a rejection episode and may lose the transplanted face. This situation shall be life threatening. There are different immunosuppressive drugs (some available at your chemist and some other restricted for hospital use). Your doctors will decide which best suits you.

6. What are the possible complications?

The most important issue that you must understand is that during the procedure, given the different complex situations that may arise during the operation, your surgeons may decide to abort the transplant.

Other relevant complications include:

(a) *Anaesthetic complications:*

Allergic reactions, bronchospasm, shock, anaphylaxis, hypoxia, anoxic cerebral damage, cardiac arrest and death

(b) *Surgical complications:*

Massive haemorrhage: Most probably, you will receive large amounts of blood products (transfusion) during and after the operation. A re-intervention for bleeding problems is not uncommon.

Vascular complications: During the operation your surgeons will anastomose (stitch together) blood vessels, some of them of very small diameter (millimetres). The most common complications include thrombosis and stenosis of blood vessels. They will require a re-intervention.

Other possible complications include bleeding, massive haemorrhage, infection, tissue necrosis (death of tissues), necrosis of the transplanted face (death of the transplant) and death. Any other complication that may occur during plastic surgery operations, craniomaxillofacial procedures or transplant surgery may occur. Other complications include common complications of other surgeries such as deep vein thrombosis and massive lung embolism.

(c) *Medical complications:*

In some cases of acute and severe rejection, it may be necessary to remove the transplanted face. You will be initially cared for in the intensive care unit (mechanical ventilation, nasogastric tubes, drains, central lines and urinary bladder catheters). These manoeuvres favour infections derived from intensive manipulation of your veins and systems with lines and tubes (urinary, line infections; pneumonia). Other infections may be caused by the depression of your immune system (immunosuppression): you will be taking medications that depress your defences and you will be more prone than the normal population for the development and to acquire viral or fungal infections. These infections may be lethal and you will be asked to take medications to prevent them.

Acute rejection: This may develop days or months after the transplant. The risk decreases months and years after the transplant, although it may still develop or chronic rejection may appear. Rejection is a common complication and it may lead to transplant failure and the need to remove the transplanted face. Biopsies will be performed on a regular basis to monitor rejection (initially every week).

Medication side effects: renal insufficiency, diabetes, neurotoxicity, high blood pressure, lipid alterations, infections, hepatic disease, etc.; sometimes these complications force to change the dose or the type of the medications.

Less common but possible complications include the transmission of infections or the reproduction of tumours (if they were removed before the transplant in the donor) or the development of new malignant tumours; of note is the development of lymphatic tumours.

7. Other important information/considerations

In order to warrant your survival and to prevent any side effects or adverse events of medications, you will have to attend our clinic for the rest of your life. These visits will include blood test and interview with the different face team members. Your doctors will modify or/ and adapt the visits and the drugs depending on every situation.

Your doctors are the only persons allowed to perform any change in the medication regime or the dose of the medication. You must not change the medications or the dosage on your own. If you do not take your medications or change them without the supervision of your doctor, it may lead to transplant failure and a life-threatening condition.

Mr./Mrs. ……………………………………

Passport/National Identity Number:………….

Expresses that:

I have been informed by the face transplant team regarding all risks and benefits of the treatment proposed to me and that I do accept to be operated on and receive a face transplantation.

I have understood all risks and possible complications that may occur. I have had the opportunity to ask any questions I deemed appropriate and that they have been answered in a comprehensive manner and that I understood them.

Consequently hereby, by signing this informed consent, I voluntarily accept and authorise this procedure.

Signed by the doctor and the patient, with date and place.

Abstract

The process of donation, including the selection of donors and transplant coordination, is an extremely relevant issue in the success of VCA programmes and in the final functional and aesthetic outcome in face transplantation. A multiple organ donation is expected, with stable haemodynamic status, although there is no contraindication for the utilisation of vasopressors. The face tissues are extremely well vascularised; thus, priority should be paid to the maintenance of good perfusion to internal organs.

The process of donation, including the selection of donors and transplant coordination, is an extremely relevant issue in the success of VCA programmes and in the final functional and aesthetic outcome in face transplantation. A multiple organ donation is expected, with stable haemodynamic status, although there is no contraindication for the utilisation of vasopressors. The face tissues are extremely well vascularised; thus, priority should be paid to the maintenance of good perfusion to internal organs.

There are different specific issues that must be taken into consideration, which makes donation in composite tissues much more difficult than solid organ transplantation. As in any other solid organ transplant process, any biological parameter must be evaluated and matched to obtain good outcomes. For optimal results, many other considerations must be taken into account: skin colour, anatomical landmarks, gender, race, age and anthropomorphic information/measurements.

The latter is very relevant, the face and the structures to be transplanted have a three-dimensional fashion in special the bones of the face skeleton and similar structures should be sought. A perfect match between face donor structures and those found in the recipient is the final goal of the donor evaluation. The same measurements that were performed in the recipient during the evaluation process should be explored in every donor that may appear during the search (Table 7.1).

Every effort should be made to obtain X-ray imaging, although the circumstances of the patient (intensive therapy unit [ITU] admission, haemodynamic instability, other injuries, etc.) may not allow transportation of the patient to the radiology department. Transplant coordinators are involved in the whole process of donation and transplantation; in those patients, especially those affected of traumatic head injury, that are transferred to the department for their injuries, a face

Table 7.1 Required anthropomorphic clinical measurements for donor matching

1. Interpupillary distance
2. Intercanthal (external) distance
3. Head perimeter (brow level)
4. Hairline–nasion distance
5. Nasal length
6. Upper lip–chin distance
7. Hairline–chin distance
8. Inter-preauricular distance

CT scan should be performed to make the required measurements and matching.

Organ and tissue donation legal status differs among countries. In some countries, all citizens are considered potential donors unless they have informed on the contrary; meanwhile, in other countries only people that have expressed their will for donation will be considered as donors. In any case, VCA is considered a clinical experimental treatment, and special and individual informed consent is required. Consent for donation follows similar guidelines. Consent for organ donation does not imply consent for tissues and composite vascularised tissues. A specific consent for this type of the donation must be obtained. During the informed consent process, the donor's family and relatives have to be informed regarding the specifics of the operation, type of tissues and structures that will be transplanted and the results of such donation in the body of the donor.

Vascularised composite tissue allotransplantation is not invisible (Fig. 7.1). Non-vascularised tissue donation is much more difficult than organ donation. Society is not as conscious as with solid organs of the real necessity of these tissues (corneas, skin, blood vessels, bones, etc.) for the general health and the recovery of some diseases. When it comes to VCA donation, the issue is much more problematic: it is not longer a question of plain tissue donation from hidden anatomic parts, but a donation of parts of the body, fully comparable to solid organs. The real difference is that VCA donation is no longer "invisible". Faces or limbs will be removed with its consequences on the mourning and presentation of the cadaver. It is mandatory to perform a prosthetic reconstruction of the cadaver (face masks or limb prosthesis) to

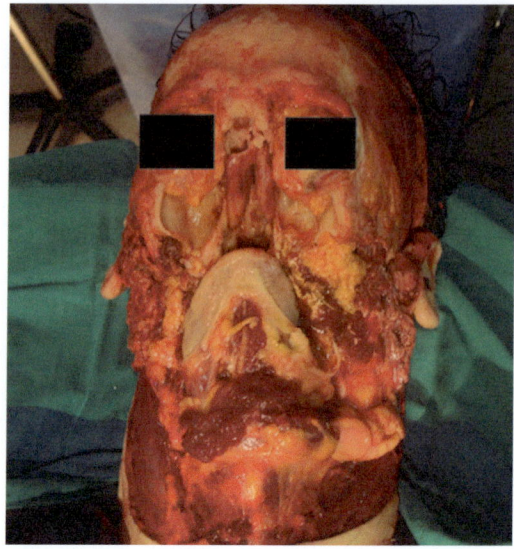

Fig. 7.1 Typical appearance of face procurement in a fresh cadaver anatomical dissection. The common results after this operation prevents any cadaver presentation

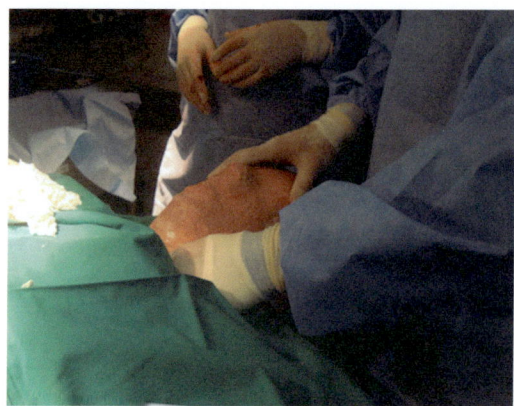

Fig. 7.2 Ethics during face VCA procurement. Fabrication of custom-made face prosthesis restores the dignity of the donor. It is compulsory in all face transplantation programmes

provide dignity to the donation process and release the body in the best possible appearance (Fig. 7.2). Donor' relatives are informed of all these special issues in VCA donation and are requested to sign an individualised informed consent that covers all the relevant information on tissue donation, consequences on the donor, type of expected defect, face structures that will be transplanted and type of restoration.

7.1 Inclusion and Exclusion Criteria for Face Donation

The overall face donation process is included within the whole coordination for donation of organs and tissues. Transplant coordinators are specialised doctors from different services (more commonly anaesthesiologists and intensive care physicians) that work full time for the coordination of organ and tissue transplantation during a period of their professional life. During the active search for donors, the coordinators check every single possible donor that matches the specific requirements for the recipient. The donor is first evaluated as any patient considered for transplantation of solid organs (tissue typing, infections, serology, etc), and those that pass the initial triage as potential donors are then evaluated for VCA.

7.1.1 Inclusion Criteria

1. Multiorgan donor with diagnosis of brain death
2. Signed informed consent from relatives for the procurement of face tissues
3. Compatibility of
   (a) Age
   (b) Gender (if applicable)
   (c) Skin tone (if applicable)
   (d) Age
   (e) Blood group (ABO) and rhesus compatible
4. Morphometric measurements, height and weight similar to recipient

Donor selection parameters may seem very specific at first, although some of them are general guidelines for the selection of potential donors of face VCA. It is extremely difficult to match perfectly all parameters (age, height, weight and measurements), but perfect and excellent function and aesthetic outcomes shall be obtained with an approximation to these parameters. The surgeon-in-chief and surgeon's team will make the final decision regarding final compatibility of the donor. The type of tissues and structures that shall be transplanted differ among recipients; it is individualised and the transplant specimen will be different from one patient to another. Therefore, the informed consent is individual for each donation. There is a tendency in many groups, though, to procure a full-face specimen and discard on the recipient the parts that will not be transplanted eventually.

7.1.2 Exclusion Criteria

All donors are evaluated conforming to all requirements of the local, regional and national tissue and organ transplantation legal bodies. All donors are evaluated as potential multiorgan donors and all inclusion and exclusion criteria apply.

In addition to that, there are specific exclusion criteria for face donation:
- Sepsis and septic shock
- HIV
- Hepatitis B and/or C
- Viral encephalitis
- Malignant neoplasms
- Active intravenous drug abuse
- Tattoos performed in the last 6 months
- Face paralysis
- Peripheral hereditary neuropathy
- Infectious or inflammatory peripheral neuropathies
- Systemic infections with associated neuropathies
- Toxic neuropathies
- Neurological neoplasms
- Rheumatoid arthritis
- Autoimmune diseases
- Diseases of collagen
- Acute face trauma
- Presence of face deformity
- Positive MRSA and other multiple resistance microorganisms

The former list is extensive but does not exclude any other significant disease or condition that may be encountered during the evaluation process. The face transplant team evaluates the donor after all the information has been gathered and takes into consideration any deformity, disease, condition to accept or decline the donor based on all the information available and the condition, urgency and match with the recipient.

7.2   Clinical Evaluation and Coordination with Transplant Donation

Transplantation of vascularised face composite tissues has relevant implications in the donation (Fig. 7.3) and in the transplantation process (Table 7.2). Composite allotransplantation programmes emerge in the transplantation world and have to adapt to a well-designed and organised model of multiorgan procurement and transplantation. Coordinators need to implement the donation of visible vascularised tissues in the donation model. Tissue donation is much more complicated than the rest of the organs; society understands the necessity of vital organs for the survival of people with failure of vital organs. However, the knowledge of the necessity for donation of tissues is poor although it

---

Implications in the donation process:

- Tissue donation much more complicated then rest of organs
- FCTA not invisible
- Cadaver presentation not possible
- Important psychosocial impact on relatives
- Possibility of a negative effect on the overall organ donation process
- Non-vital therapy

Hospital Universitari Vall d'Hebron

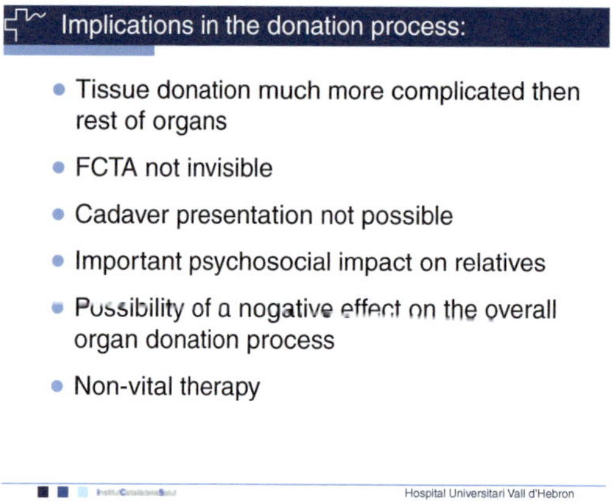

Fig. 7.3 The implications of face donation are very relevant and could have negative effects in the overall donation process. Vital solid organs always have priority

Table 7.2 Implications in the donation process

Multiple organ donation expected
Important impact on the rest of transplantation teams
Thoracic, heart, multivisceral surgeons
Exhaustive coordination involved
Longer overall donation time
Ethics in the treatment of the donor

serves for the improvement of quality of life in some patients and for the survival after severe diseases. Moreover, there is a fear for the visibility of tissue donation, and an intensive interview is necessary to obtain the donation of tissues. Face and limbs have also an emotional impact; thus, donation is extremely difficult. The impact that donation of the face and limbs may have on relatives has to be taken into account, and extreme care has to be implemented during the donation interview. VCA is in general terms a nonvital therapy; it aims at improvements in quality of life. Consequently, during the donation process, all team members must remember that the first priority is successful internal vital solid organ donation. When team members implement a programme of VCA, they have to make sure that this process is maintained and that face and limb allotransplantation does not have a negative impact on the overall donation process. The initial experiences throughout the world have been extremely positive. The process has not had any negative effect, and all programmes have received a positive feedback from society.

In order to optimise face VCA, donation and to overcome all possible negative effects of face donation, the VCA team and the coordination of donation and transplantation at the Vall d'Hebron University Hospital developed a specific protocol for this type of transplantation. The request for face donation (or other VCA donations: hands, legs, etc.) may have an important emotional impact on relatives. This type of request is ordinarily performed at a time of intense psychosocial stress: a sudden event in the health biography of a close relative (spouse, parents, or children) has had the outcome of death (brain death) and the request for donation of internal organs. Relatives are very fragile during this period and all efforts must be made to make the transition as smooth as possible with full psychosocial support. The request for face donation in all donors that were compatible in biological terms could harm relatives and the overall donation process. Therefore, since many of the possible donors may be discarded by the transplant team due to skin tone, morphometric

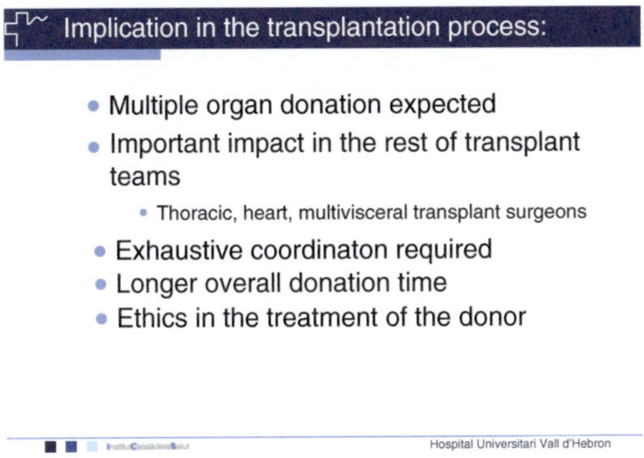

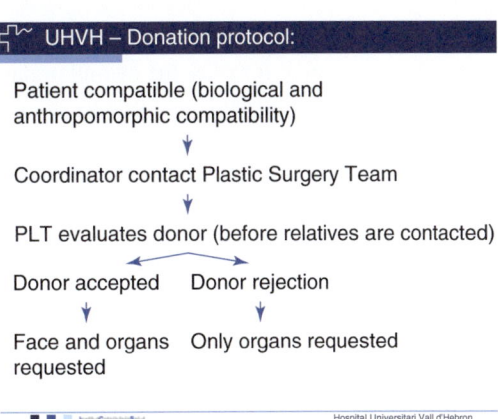

Implication in the transplantation process:

- Multiple organ donation expected
- Important impact in the rest of transplant teams
  - Thoracic, heart, multivisceral transplant surgeons
- Exhaustive coordinaton required
- Longer overall donation time
- Ethics in the treatment of the donor

InstitutCatalàdelaSalut   Hospital Universitari Vall d'Hebron

Fig. 7.4 Multiple organ donations in young patients are expected. A team approach is mandatory

UHVH – Donation protocol:

Patient compatible (biological and anthropomorphic compatibility)

↓

Coordinator contact Plastic Surgery Team

↓

PLT evaluates donor (before relatives are contacted)

Donor accepted   Donor rejection

↓   ↓

Face and organs   Only organs requested
requested

InstitutCatalàdelaSalut   Hospital Universitari Vall d'Hebron

Fig. 7.5 The UHVH donation protocol intends to minimise the psychological impact of face VCA donation request

measurements, skin quality or many other issues, a specific protocol for face donation was developed to limit the number of face donation requests (Fig. 7.4). Transplant coordinators follow the clinical course and hospital course of any patient that present with a rapid and profound deterioration of Glasgow Coma Score (GSC). They are not involved in the clinical treatment of patients whatsoever. Patients that continue to deteriorate and have initial signs or symptoms of irreversible cerebral damage enter the initial laboratory evaluation and medical history evaluation to rule out any contraindications. All clinical efforts continue to improve the clinical picture of the patient and treat him/her accordingly to have a good final outcome. However, despite all clinical efforts, some patients continue to deteriorate and a diagnosis of brain death is finally reached. The face transplant team is contacted if a patient is deemed to be compatible to any of the recipients in the waiting list for face transplantation. The surgeon evaluates the patients and determines whether the donor is a good match for the recipient. If a match is reached, the coordinators start the donation protocol with the request for solid organs and VCA donations. If the VCA team refuses the donor, coordinators request donation for solid organs and tissues without face or other VCA request for donation. This protocol has proved to be extremely effective to obtain a good positive return of donations, both for VCA and solid organs, limiting the emotional stress

and possible negative effect of the VCA request for donation (Fig. 7.5).

The implications of VCA programmes are no less cumbersome than the donation process. A multiple organ donation is expected. The best candidate donors are selected for face VCA donation; thus, all solid organs and tissues are considered for transplantation. A longer operative time during procurement is expected and an exhaustive and intense preparation and coordination among all transplant teams is mandatory. Thoracic organ procurement shall be involved, and liver, lungs and heart optimal procurement is a must. It is highly advised that during the preparation for a VCA programme, the face VCA team get to know all the issues involved in multiple organ donation and be involved in different procurements to get used to the timing and procedures that are normally performed. It is also imperative that some important parts of the procedure are planned together with the rest of the teams, such as the need for tracheotomy (in case of a double lung transplantation) and the timing of face procurement. This may vary among VCA teams. Some have performed procurement at the beginning of the operation, some others together with the rest of teams and some others at the end of the procurement without active circulation. The latter has the risk of a longer ischaemia time and risk of massive haemorrhage during reperfusion. We advise the procurement in a heart-beating donor. It makes the overall organisation much more difficult but follows all the tenets of optimal organ procurement: in situ dissection, correct haemostasis and short ischaemia time. In our hands, simultaneous procurement of the face tissues together with in situ dissection of abdominal organs proved to be safe, shortens the operative time and allows for a team approach. Before the procedure, a face impression should be obtained (see Fig. 7.2). Face impression can be obtained in the ITU when the donor has been accepted and is being prepared for the procurement. Conversely, the impression can be obtained in the operative theatre before the operation starts. During the procurement, a face mask (resin or silicone custom-made face prosthesis) is fashioned, and it is applied to the head in order to preserve dignity and follow ethics during the procurement. This issue is mandatory in all VCA protocols, and it must be stated so in the ethics submission. The mask is trimmed and fixated during the closure of all incisions (thoracic and abdominal incisions).

7.3   Appendix 7.1: Informed Consent for the Donation of Face Allograft

Information that family and relatives of the donor must receive and understand:

1. You are being asked to donate the face structures of your relative (listed in section 3) for the transplantation of the face or parts of the face to reconstruct the face structures of a recipient (patient with severe face deformity). The recipient has been evaluated in a comprehensive manner by the face transplantation team and all reconstructive options have been taken into account. The transplantation of a full or partial face has remained the last and only option to reconstruct the face of the recipient. The face transplant team has proposed to utilise…*(list the parts of the face)*…of the face of another person (the donor).

2. The goals of this surgical intervention (the face transplantation) are:
    (a) Obtain a cosmetically acceptable face appearance.
    (b) Improve his/her quality of life.
    (c) Reassume a normal personal and social life interaction.
3. Apart from the internal organs (your transplant coordinator has informed you about solid organ donation separately), the following structures of the face will be obtained:
    (a) *List all that apply.*
    (b) *(…)*
4. The face appearance of the donor will not be maintained in the recipient after face transplantation. The aesthetics and face appearance depend on the face skeleton or part of it if bones are also transplanted. A new identity will be created, not resembling at all whatsoever the appearance of the donor.
5. Following the donation and procurement of the donor's face or part of it, the face transplant team shall make every effort to restore the appearance of the donor by means of a custom-made face prosthesis, in order to preserve the dignity of the donor. You should anticipate, though, that the presentation of the cadaver will no longer be possible.
6. The face transplant team and all health workers involved in the donation and transplantation will preserve the intimacy of the donor's and recipient's family and shall make every effort to maintain their anonymous identity.
7. The medical team will publicly announce the face transplantation few days after the transplant has been completed in order to stimulate donations, to improve the knowledge of face deformity in society and to help future recipients and relatives for future transplantations.
8. The medical team involved in face transplantation does not receive any economic compensation by this type of reconstruction:

Signed,
Name and surname:
Relationship with donor:
Date:

7.4   Appendix 7.2: Legal Diligence for VCA Donation

Deceased personal details (name, date of birth, address):

....

Details of the person(s) giving informed consent (list all that apply):

Name in full:

Personal relationship with the deceased person:

Address:

Telephone number:

Declare:

- The absence of express opposition of the deceased person to donate the face after his/her death to be transplanted to another person that may need it
- That I/we have been informed that the medical team that will carry out the face transplantation will make a custom-made mask and that they will apply this prosthesis on the deceased head and that they have informed me/us that donor's appearance will not be recognisable in the recipient's new face.

Signature of the person(s) making the declaration

Date

General Medical Support in Face Transplantation

8

Abstract

Postoperative care of composite tissue allotransplantation patients has significant differences when compared to other solid organ transplantation procedures. In general terms, the management of these types of patients is less complex than solid organ transplantation; however, some specific issues complicate it, including immunological barriers, antigen load of composite tissues, surgical stress, and bleeding and fluid management.

Postoperative care of composite tissue allotransplantation patients has significant differences when compared to other solid organ transplantation procedures. In general terms, the management of these types of patients is less complex than solid organ transplantation; however, some specific issues complicate it:

1. Immunological barriers
2. Antigen load of composite tissues
3. Surgical stress
4. Bleeding and fluid management

As in any other transplant discipline, VCA is performed across the major histocompatibility complex. Still, antigenicity of composite tissues and skin is considered to be much higher than any other solid organ. Shortage of compatible donors (both biological and morphological) makes tissue type matching almost impossible. HLA mismatch is common among recipients, and immunosuppression regimens need to be intense. Patients will require a multidisciplinary support to obtain the desired outcome, and sig-nificant surveillance is necessary to avoid side effects and complications.

Face transplantation is an aggressive and long surgical intervention. Duration varies, and recipient's operative time has been reported between 15 and 30 h. During the procedure different techniques are combined (soft tissues resections, craniomaxillofacial and microsurgical techniques); the operation begins with the resection of deformed and scarred tissues, preparation of blood vessels and nerves, trimming of bony segments and osteotomies for correct skeletal alignment. It is followed by the reconstruction of the defect with a composite tissue allotransplantation (the face allograft). Revascularisation has been performed in different time sequences, although it is recommended to perform revascularisation at the early stages of VCA, in order to minimise ischaemia–reperfusion injury. The combination of different techniques in this complex reconstruction makes massive blood loss a common scenario. The surgical team should be prepared to prevent and treat appropriately important haemorrhages. Fluid management should be titrated to response, and all necessary preparations for the early postoperative period are prepared in order to avoid complications.

Still, composite tissue allotransplantation is an elective surgery procedure, which can be prepared ahead on time; recipients are normally healthy patients that do not present with organ or system dysfunctions or failure. Hence, it is considered to be a safe transplant surgery discipline that provides good outcomes provided a robust team approach is implemented. Patients are admitted to the surgical intensive care unit for postoperative management. Fluid management, enteral nutrition, immunosuppression, respiratory support, wound care and microsurgical postoperative control are necessary.

During the early postoperative period, patients may develop problems and complications caused by different conditionings, which include:

(a) Organ and system deterioration/dysfunction
(b) Intensive/aggressive critical-care support
(c) Immunosuppression

Operative time has a direct impact on morbidity and complications. Long operations, massive blood transfusions, aggressive fluid replacement and respiratory infections impact systems and organ function. A critical-care holistic approach to minimise the impact of surgical stress and organ support must be implemented in order to obtain a good transition and excellent outcomes. One should not obviate that aggressive respiratory support, broad-spectrum antibiotics, immunosuppression and other interventions may produce side effects and complications. They require judicious and rigorous management and state-of-the-art nursing to prevent complications. Patients may also present with infections and acute rejection episodes, although they may be not as frequent as in other type of solid organ transplantation. In addition, acute rejection episodes do not affect the function of any vital transplanted organ (like liver, kidney, lung or heart allograft) and allow for evaluation and for a careful decision-making process (avoiding important side or toxic effects of immunosuppressive agents).

8.1 General Postoperative Support

Patients are normally admitted to the surgical intensive care unit for immediate postoperative care. In our scenario, patients are admitted to the burn intensive care unit, where they are provided with a protected environment with positive laminar flow, a robust team with physicians well versed in critical medicine support, control of microsurgical free flaps and nursing for complex plastic surgery operations (Fig. 8.1). Each team should review the positive and negative key elements for postoperative stay in different units and choose the process that best suits for a good outcome in terms of excellence in critical support, infection control and nursing (see Appendix 8.1 for specific information).

Patients are admitted to the intensive care intubated and ventilated. Our clinical protocol includes an elective tracheotomy (if not already present) for correct and safe management of the airway and quick respiratory weaning. Patients

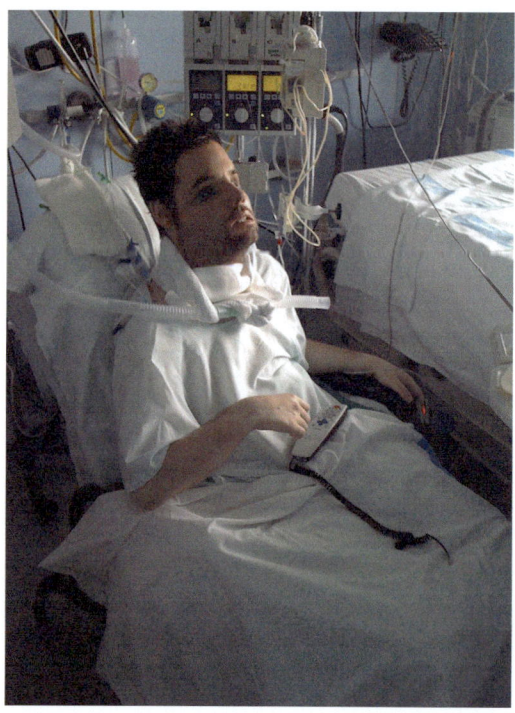

Fig. 8.1 Good postoperative nursing and critical care are key issues for correct outcomes in face VCA

are waken up and wean off the ventilator as soon as the patient is haemodynamically stable, recovers a good core temperature and does not show any sign of respiratory failure or any other organ/system dysfunction. We recommend to keep the patient sedated overnight if surgery is completed after hours, although every effort should be made to wean off the patient as soon as possible to avoid any respiratory complication.

Patients are fed through an enteral route either after weaning or with an early enteral feeding protocol if patients are not awake right after the operation. Depending on the type of deformity and the functional impact of the missing anatomy, patients will have a gastrostomy tube in place. All other patients receive enteral nutrition via an NG or NJ tube. The team should evaluate the type of transplant that is being proposed and the expected initial functional impact on swallowing and oral competence. If surgeons expect a longer postoperative time to start oral feeding, one should consider a percutaneous gastrostomy tube placement. Extreme care should be implemented in patients that are fed through a nasal tube. The transplanted nose is insensate, protective sensation may not be present until the second to third months post transplant and it will improve overtime. Therefore, patients are at risk for the development of a pressure sore on the nose (similarly to those seen in paediatric/neonatal ulcerations). Padding and protection is mandatory if the nasal route is utilised, and it should be discontinued as soon as the patient can reassume oral feeding. Invasive monitoring is maintained for as long as the patient requires haemodynamic drugs; it should be discontinued thereafter to avoid complications and infections. Central lines are nursed with extreme care to avoid line sepsis and/or phlebitis. Every effort should be made for an early removal, mandated by intravenous (IV) medication (in special systemic antibiotic prophylaxis and immunosuppression).

An aggressive rehabilitation protocol is implemented, with early passive and active range of motion, active aerobic exercise and walking. All patients should be actively encouraged to walk and exercise in order to maintain muscle tone and function. Specific rehabilitation professionals include face paralysis physiotherapists and speech pathology specialists. They start the physiotherapy protocol in the early phase, and it is continued over time for as long as the expected final functional outcome is achieved.

8.1.1   Nutritional Support

Composite tissue allotransplantation patients are healthy individuals that do not present organ failures or dysfunction before the transplant. Most of the patients are fed orally with a normal diet unless the deformity prevents so. Still, nutritional status in the pre-transplant phase should be considered normal.

Surgical stress, immunosuppression, medications and acute rejections significantly affect nutritional status and trigger a catabolic hypermetabolic response. It is necessary to maintain a well-balanced nutritional status and body weight. Acute rejections and other complications and side effects may have a relevant impact on all systems; thus, a strong physiological reserve will help to overcome these events and prolong long-term survival.

Immediately after surgery the patients are kept nil by mouth for 24 h with the exception of oral medications. In the second postoperative day, enteral nutrition via a nasojejunal tube or gastrostomy is started. Enteral nutrition is prolonged for 10 days; patients start then an oral intake for liquids and progress to a soft diet and normal diet in the following days unless dictated otherwise by the postoperative progress of patients. As soon as the patient can maintain his/her caloric requirements, enteral nutrition is discontinued completely. General principles of nutritional support are listed in Table 8.1. A re-evaluation of nutritional status after admission is mandatory; the patient's nutritional background is determined and chronic conditions, recent weight changes and nutritional preferences noted (Table 8.2). Intolerance to enteral nutrition, including diarrhoea, may be produced by many causes, although a team member should remember that one of the most common aetiologies for intolerance and diarrhoea is infection and sepsis. VCA patients

Table 8.1 General principles of nutritional support in VCA

All transplant patients must receive an adequate nutrition as soon as possible
Parenteral nutrition should be used only when enteral nutrition fails
Caloric requirements are determined by indirect calorimetry (enteral formulas may be used as an alternative)
Limit protein intake in renal impairment
Prevent weight loss; it is very difficult to regain body composition
List all intake in nutritional sheet
Adopt an early enteral feeding protocol
Offer milk and juices
Maintain oral nutritional supplements during hospital admission
Do not use opioids during meals
Perform a nutritional background evaluation on admission and control nutritional status twice a week

Table 8.2 Initial nutritional control

Weight and height
Lymphocyte count
Total leukocyte count
Haemoglobin and haematocrit
Erythrocyte mean corpuscular volume
Albumin, pre-albumin, magnesium, phosphate, calcium (ion), copper, zinc, protoporphyrin/haemoglobin, vitamin D, folic acid
24 h nitrogen
Indirect calorimetry

Incidence of viral infections, such as cytomegalovirus (CMV) and Epstein–Barr virus (EPV), should be similar to that observed in low-risk SOT (kidney transplantation). Prevention of infection against CMV and EPV and *Pneumocystis jirovecii* is delivered following the renal transplantation protocol (see Chap. 9).

are immunosuppressed, and as such patients may not exhibit the full spectrum of signs and symptoms of impending sepsis. Infection may follow a more insidious initial phase; hence, suspicion and prompt treatment is necessary.

8.1.3   Immunosuppression

The main objectives of immunosuppressive treatments include maintenance of correct graft function, absence of acute and chronic rejection, achievement of graft tolerance and the avoidance or minimisation of potential toxic or side effects of medications. Strategies for the modulation of the immune response in transplantation medicine can be divided into two main phases or stages: the induction and the maintenance immunosuppression. The whole face transplantation team must be well versed in all types of immunosuppression, timing for treatment and potential risks and side effects. Induction therapy begins in the preoperative period, and it is continued during revascularisation and immediate postoperative care.

8.1.2   Infection Control

There are few significant differences between VCA and solid organ transplantation (SOT) that make infection both extremely relevant and a challenging venture:

1. VCA requires initial doses of immunosuppression significantly higher than SOT.
2. VCA are non-sterile grafts (the skin is exposed to the environment, different amounts of mucosa are involved, sinuses and teeth are included in the graft), although the lymphoid load of the grafts is not very high.
3. There is limited experience in infection control protocols and long-term outcomes of VCA.

In general terms, bacterial infection prophylaxis should contemplate prevention of infections in the oral and maxillofacial area. Therefore, prophylaxis includes oral bacterial flora for donors with an intensive care unit stay of more than 48 h.

8.1.3.1 Induction Therapy
The objective of the initial phase is to achieve an intense immunosuppression during the first week post transplant in order to reduce the probability of early acute rejection. In general terms, induction therapy is performed by the intravenous infusion of a monoclonal or polyclonal antibody, which tends to reduce the severity of any rejection

episode and favours the development of long-term tolerance. During this induction period, maintenance therapy is started and monitored to adjust the doses of drugs to the serum target and the clinical response.

8.1.3.2 Maintenance Therapy

The scope of this immunosuppression protocol consists in a strategy to suppress the recipient's immunological response against the allograft, inhibiting their ability to recognise the foreign tissues and to organise an orchestrated response. The drug regimen is adapted on an individual basis to reach the minimal doses of medications that allows for a correct immunomodulation with minimal toxicity. Immune adaptation allows for decreasing doses of medications over time while maintaining the same effect. A treatment regimen that employs multiple drugs produces a synergistic and adjunctive effect of immunosuppression minimising toxicities.

Our current immunosuppression protocol at the University Hospital Vall d'Hebron is based on a three-drug regime and induction with Thymoglobulin and prednisone.

Induction Therapy

1. Preoperative infusion of Thymoglobulin (atg) as soon as the patient arrives to the hospital, at a dose of 2 mg/kg. Premedicate with 1 g of methylprednisolone IV, Benadryl 50 mg IV and acetaminophen 650 mg PO.
2. Revascularisation: Administer 1 g of methylprednisolone IV, 30 min before revascularisation.
3. Thymoglobulin (atg) 2 mg/kg/day for 5 days (start preoperatively)
4. Methylprednisolone:
   - Days 1–14: Administer a dose of 2 mg/kg/day.
   - Taper down the dose of methylprednisolone over time to 10 mg/day.
5. Tacrolimus 0.15 mg/kg/day divided in two doses. Start treatment preoperatively.
6. Mycophenolate mofetil. Initial dose of 1 g two times a day (total dose of 2 g). Start preoperatively. Adjust to leukocyte count and stop 1 year after the transplant.

Maintenance Therapy

1. Tacrolimus: Serum target levels of 10–15 ng/ml during the first 6 months (months 1–6 post transplant) and target levels of 5–10 ng/ml after month 6 post transplant.
2. Mycophenolate mofetil: Adjust levels to leukocyte count.
3. Methylprednisolone: Taper down levels to 10 mg/day. Consider lower levels or alternate levels if good response.
4. Topical tacrolimus 0.1 % 2 times/day during 2 months (start on day 10 post transplant).

Patients are monitored on a daily basis for side effects of the treatment and blood levels in order to adjust the immunosuppression regime and achieve the minimal dosage that maintains good function and graft tolerance without signs of rejection.

8.2   Management of Complications in Face VCA

Face transplantation is one of the most complex operations that exist to date. It combines the risks and complexity of solid organ transplantation, reconstructive microsurgery, major tissue resection and reconstruction and craniomaxillofacial techniques. However, excellent outcomes have been obtained so far, with a low mortality rate (0 % intraoperative, 4 % immediate postoperative, 8 % long-term mortality rate, approximately), which supports the beneficial effects of a robust team approach. There have been few experiences worldwide in face VCA; thus, the real long-term outcome and survival rate are still to be defined.

The most frequent complication can be divided, as in any other surgical discipline, into two main groups:
(a) Surgical complications
(b) Medical or nonsurgical complications

Complications of surgery may be encountered directly during the operative procedure or more commonly in the immediate postoperative period, being less common in the chronic long-term phase of VCA. Medical complications can occur anytime from the induction phase of immunosuppression to the whole process of convalescence and chronic long-term phase. The prevalence of the latter complication increases as time elapses.

8.2.1 Surgical Complications

These types of complications do not differ much from other problems that are commonly encountered during reconstructive surgery that includes microsurgical tissue transfer and craniomaxillofacial techniques. The most common surgical complications are normally managed with good outcomes by the plastic surgery team involved in face transplantation. As mentioned before, they do not differ much from similar complications encountered in other plastic surgery patients, and they include:

- Arterial or venous thrombosis (microvascular pedicle)
- Wound dehiscence
- Partial necrosis (skin or skin/adipose tissue)
- Bleeding, haemorrhage/haematoma
- Failure of VCA caused by non-salvage thrombosis
- Soft tissue infections/abscesses

Management of surgical complications do not differ much from medical and surgical management of complications encountered in reconstructive microsurgery. Surgical techniques include revision of microanastomosis, correct wound care and correction of wound dehiscence, utilisation of grafts and flaps, abscess and other collection drainage and correct haemostasis. One must bear in mind, though, that any surgical intervention during the postoperative period has to follow strict protocol guidelines regarding infection control, management of tissues and maintenance of immunosuppression. Antibiotic prophylaxis is a must. Infection control team members should be consulted and systemic antibiotics be administered to prevent surgical site infection and systemic dissemination. Immunosuppression has to be continued and close monitored during the postoperative period to adjust the drug dose if necessary. Fasting periods and IV fluids may alter the homeostasis and the medication levels. Medications are titrated to response, allowing a quick and rejection free recovery.

Similarly to any plastic surgery reoperation, good care of tissues is mandatory. Skin and soft tissue necrosis and/or wound dehiscence would compromise patient recovery and increase the risk for progressive graft failure and invasive infection.

8.2.2 Medical Complications

Nonsurgical complications and adverse events in the VCA patient are diverse and may be divided into acute medical complications and adverse events of general care and immunosuppression. The latter are similar to the transplantation population.

8.2.2.1 Acute Medical Complications
Preservation Injury
This is the first histopathological finding in any solid organ transplantation. Prolonged ischaemia time and ischaemia–reperfusion injury play a principal role in this situation. This is a minor problem in face VCA. All transplanted tissues in VCA have low metabolic rate and may sustain a prolonged ischaemia time. Cumulative experience in reconstructive microsurgery and hand and limb reimplantation sustains this clinical evidence. However, as in any other transplant discipline, reperfusion should be started as soon as possible in order to prevent any preservation injury.

Rejection Episodes
This is the most frequent acute medical complication in face VCA. Data extracted from the international hand registry indicate that approximately 85 % of all VCA recipients (including the face, hand, limbs and others) develop at least one acute rejection episode. Face tissues do not carry with a high amount of lymphoid tissues. The skin, mucosa and soft tissues, though, may produce a strong immune response, and it is not uncommon to suffer two or even three rejection episodes in face allograft recipients (Figs. 8.2 and 8.3). During the immediate postoperative period, the induction immunosuppression therapy is continued with decreasing doses of corticoids, aiming to achieve maintenance therapy in a short course of time. Tacrolimus is started on day 1 and

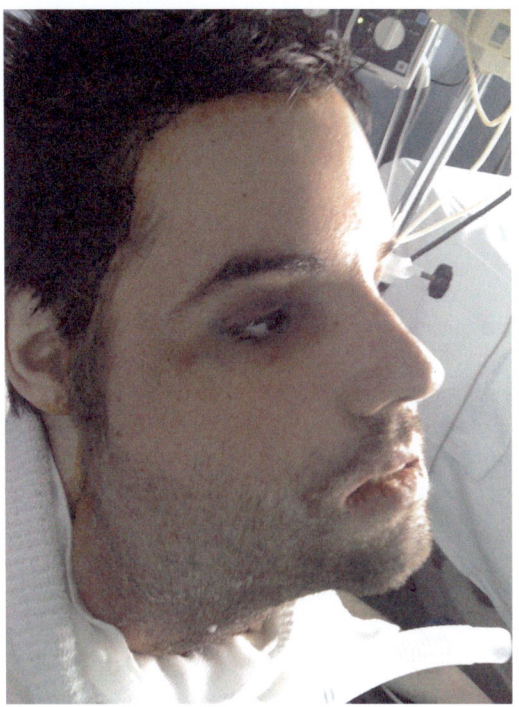

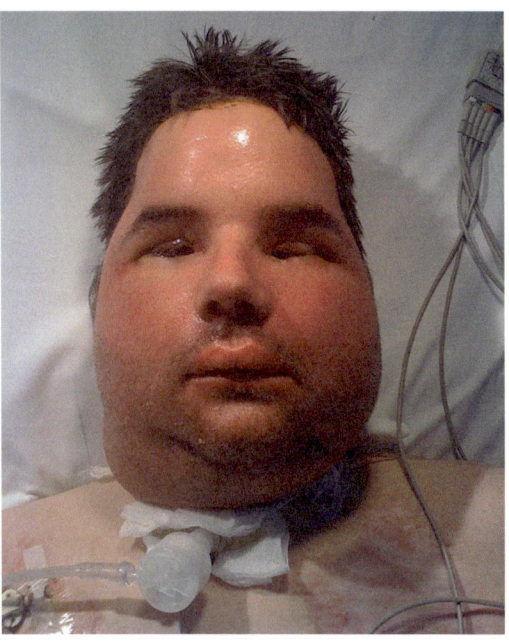

Fig. 8.3 Same patient 7 days afterwards; note the intense oedema and erythematous appearance during an acute rejection episode (grade II–III)

Fig. 8.2 Typical appearance of a full-face transplantation recipient at 3 weeks after the transplant

blood levels are monitored on a daily basis with target through levels of 10–15 ug/ml for the first 6 months after the face transplantation. The patient is inspected every day to detect any changes in face appearance and any signs of rejection. We strongly advise daily photographic evaluation that allows for retrospective analysis of the physical exploration since rejection signs develop slowly.

The diagnosis of any acute rejection episode is reached by a combination of clinical inspection and histopathological confirmation in skin and mucosal biopsies. A positive biopsy for acute rejection without clinical signs and symptoms is only informative. The clinical scenario should always confirm the diagnosis. Close follow-up is advised in case of histopathological signs of rejection in an asymptomatic patient. Excessive immunosuppression carries with a high risk for infectious and non-infectious complications.

The most frequent signs of acute rejection consist of oedema, erythema, macular reaction (mild rejection episode), maculopapular reaction (moderate rejection) or indurated plaques with or without ulceration and necrosis (severe rejection).

The confirmation of the acute rejection episode is performed by skin/mucosa biopsy. It is graded from 0 to 4 according to the BANFF classification. The absence of biochemical markers (such as those encountered in hepatic and renal transplantation) makes tissue biopsies (skin and mucosal biopsies) necessary for the confirmation of suspected acute rejections. The presence of perivascular mononuclear infiltrations or any other alteration in keratinocytes or tissue structures is not a sole indication for acute rejection. In the absence of pathological confirmation, other causes for clinical findings should be investigated.

Histopathological signs for acute rejection include:

- Mononuclear infiltration of the skin, mucosa or both
- Immunoglobulin or complement deposition
- Oedema
- Cellular necrosis
- Intimal hyperplasia
- Fibrosis

Table 8.3 Banff classification of composite tissue allo-transplantation rejection

Grade 0	Non specific changes
	No or only mild lymphocytic infiltration without involvement of the superficial dermal structures or epidermis
Grade I (mild rejection)	Superficial perivascular inflammation with involvement of superficial vessels and without involvement of overlying epidermis
Grade II (moderate rejection)	Features of grade I with involvement of the epithelium and adnexal structures
Grade III (severe rejection)	Band-like superficial dermal infiltrates with more continuous involvement of the epidermis and middle and deep perivascular infiltrates
Grade IV (necrotising rejection)	Features of grade III along with frank necrosis of the epidermis and other tissues

Indiscriminate utilisation of tissue biopsies should be avoided. They may compromise the final aesthetic result of the face graft (multiple scars). During the Banff meeting in A Coruña, Spain (Banff CTA-07), experts reached a consensus for the grading of pathological tissue rejection in VCA, incorporating five classifications grading the severity of acute rejection (Table 8.3). Tissue biopsies should be obtained from a specimen of a minimal diameter of 4 mm including the skin, dermal annexes, dermis, subcutaneous tissues and blood vessels. In case of a suspected acute rejection, biopsies should be obtained from erythematous indurated cutaneous areas. Recommended laboratory process includes haematoxylin and eosin (H&E) and periodic acid–Schiff (PAS). Depending on results and other experimental protocols, immunohistochemistry assays may include (but not limited) CD3, CD4, CD19, CD20, CD68, HLA-DR, CMV and C4d.20 and immunoglobulin deposition. Unless the clinical situation mandates otherwise (necrotising rejection, ulcers, severe functional impairment), the treatment for acute rejection is halted until a definitive diagnosis is obtained. In contrast to other solid organ transplantation, functional impairment does not affect vital functions; thus, definitive treatment

can be temporised. On the other hand, intense over-immunosuppression may alter or have a significant impact on other organs and systems and produce toxic levels or chronic side effects.

First line of acute rejection therapy in VCA consists of high doses of glucocorticoids (they are normally steroid sensitive) and an optimisation of the immunosuppression regime. In some cases, though, monoclonal or polyclonal antibodies may be necessary when no responses or a partial response is obtained with intravenous boluses of corticoids. When the rejection episode is limited to the skin, topical steroids or topical tacrolimus creams may be indicated. Extracorporeal phototherapy has also been proposed to diminish sensitisation in selected cases. The treatment of acute rejection episodes requires the utilisation of high doses of medications that affect the immune system and have profound implications in infection control and side effects. Severe acute rejections require hospital admission and prompt treatment.

All rejection episodes are commonly treated with boluses of prednisone, an increase in the daily prednisone dosage and optimisation of treatment:

1. Increase the dose of tacrolimus if serum blood level <15 ng/ml.
2. Methylprednisolone 1 g/day/IV for 3 days.
3. If severe rejection, methylprednisolone 5 mg/kg IV in 4 doses with quick taper over 5 days.
4. Consider topical tacrolimus and steroids.
5. Steroid-resistant rejection:
   (a) OKT3 5 mg/day/iv for 7 days or
   (b) Thymoglobulin (atg) 2 mg/kg/day for 3 days

In repeated severe acute rejections, consider extracorporeal photophoresis.

Infection

There is limited information and experience regarding the incidence of infection in face VCA recipients. Acute bacterial and fungal infections are uncommon, and most patients have a good postoperative recovery without infection episodes. During the subacute (up to 6 months) and chronic phase, some viral infections may occur, such as CMV reactivation (especially in CMV

Table 8.4 Common herpetic and varicella infections in transplant recipients

1. Herpes simplex:
   Noncomplicated mucocutaneous infection
   Severe mucocutaneous and visceral infection
   Meningoencephalitis
2. Varicella zoster:
   Localised in the dermatome
   Disseminated varicella or zoster infection

Table 8.5 Common CMV infections in VCA

Viral syndrome and hepatitis
Gastrointestinal disease
Pneumonitis

negative recipients) and Epstein–Barr virus (EBV). Pneumonia may occur, although current experience shows a low incidence. In any case, patients must be monitored and inspected for signs and symptoms for infectious episodes routinely.

During the acute phase, especially in the intensive care stay, patients are at risk for developing bacterial infection of the face graft and common post-transplant infections such as line sepsis, pneumonia and urinary infections. Opportunistic infection (fundamentally CMV and EPV) incidence is similar to that encountered in renal transplantation (low-risk solid organ transplantation), which requires similar type of immunosuppression.

Bacterial Infections

Empirical treatment should be started as soon as there is the clinical suspicion of a serious bacterial infection. We may differentiate graft infection and distant infections in other organs and/or systems. Infection of the face graft must be individualised. Each recipient receives different type of tissues and face structures, either intraoral, extraoral or both; the infection can be community or hospital acquired, and there may be deep abscesses. Treatment is normally dictated on a case-by-case basis; surgical debridement may be necessary in serious cases and in the presence of purulent collections. In severe cases or septic shock, empiric treatment should be initiated as soon as possible with broad-spectrum antibiotics (daptomycin and meropenem IV).

Other common bacterial infections in the transplant population include intraabdominal infections, pneumonia, IV-line sepsis and acute pyelonephritis. In all these situations, team members

need to differentiate between hospital- and community-acquired infections and infections with high severity scores or sepsis. One should always refer to the current local or institution's treatment guidelines for specific treatment.

Viral Infections

The presence of any viral infection in a VCA patient may be the consequence of high levels/ toxic levels of immunosuppression. This situation should always be explored and immunosuppression medications reduced if possible. The most common viruses encountered in VCA are herpes simplex, varicella zoster and CMV. Table 8.4 lists the most common herpes simplex and varicella zoster infections. Oral treatment is indicated to limited and benign conditions (oral acyclovir, famciclovir, valacyclovir), whereas endovenous treatment is indicated in severe cases (acyclovir). CMV infection is a common complication in the transplant population. Severe infections may trigger acute rejection episodes, have a significant impact in systems and organs and affect graft survival. Common infections in the transplant population are listed in Table 8.5. The decision-making process for CMV infection therapy is directed by viral load and the previous immunisation status of recipients. We must make a distinction between negative recipients (R–) and positive recipients (R+) who receive an organ from either a negative (D–) or a positive (D+) donor. In a mismatched recipient (D+/R–), all infections must be treated regardless of viral load. In all other cases (D+/R+ and D–/R+), the current advice is to treat infections with a viral antigen load >25 or more than 2,500 copies in real-time PCR. Ganciclovir and valganciclovir are the treatment of choice. The response to treatment is monitored with viral antigen load in blood samples. Treatment should be continued until a negative viral antigen load is achieved in peripheral blood.

Table 8.6 Common *Candida* spp. infections in transplant recipients

Mucosal candidiasis
Oesophageal candidiasis
Candidemia
Peritonitis
Urinary infection
Asymptomatic candiduria

Table 8.7 Side effects of immunosuppressive agents

Agent	Key adverse effects
Cyclosporine	Nephrotoxicity, neurotoxicity, hyperglycaemia, hyperlipidaemia, gingival hyperplasia, hirsutism, hypertension, malignancy
Tacrolimus	Nephrotoxicity, neurotoxicity, hyperglycaemia, gastrointestinal disturbances, hypertension, malignancy, alopecia
Corticosteroids	Hypertension, hyperglycaemia, osteoporosis, growth retardation, cataract, gastrointestinal ulceration, poor wound healing
Azathioprine	Myelosuppression, hepatotoxicity
Mycophenolic acid	Myelosuppression, gastrointestinal disturbances, malignancy
Sirolimus	Hyperlipidaemia, thrombocytopenia, anaemia, poor wound healing, pneumonitis, mucosal ulceration
Anti-lymphocyte Ab	Cytokine release phenomenon, viral activation, immune complex syndrome

Fungal Infections

Candida and *Aspergillus* infections are the most common pathogens encountered in the transplant population (Table 8.6). Face VCA may include different amounts of mucosa, tongue, face bones and sinuses. Special attention must be directed to these areas to detect initial stages of mucosal mycosis. Mucormycosis may also develop in sinuses; hence, X-ray examination and biopsies may be necessary in some circumstances. Treatment for *Candida* spp. depends on the stadium (initial, recurrent or therapeutic failure) and location. Initial phases are commonly treated orally with azoles (co-trimoxazole, fluconazole) or nystatin. Complicated cases, candidemia, peritonitis and fungal infections are treated intravenously (i.e. anidulafungin, amphotericin B).

Graft-Versus-Host Disease

Transplantation of immunocompetent donor lymph cells into an immunocompromised host may trigger a reaction of such cells against recipient's tissues, the so-called graft-versus-host disease (GVHD). This reaction occurs after the activation of specific donor cells against certain antigens of recipient's tissues. Among all organs and systems, the most commonly involved organs and tissues in GVHD are skin cells, bowel and liver. However, skin and soft tissues carry with few immunocompetent lymph cells, and the expected incidence should be extremely low. To date, no GVHD has been reported in face transplant recipients, even in those that have received donor bones as part of their transplants.

Immunosuppression Side Effects and Adverse Reactions

Immunosuppressive therapy is not risk free. Aside from the increased risk for infections, each agent can produce different adverse effects, which may be strengthened by other concomitant medications (Table 8.7). Mild to moderate side effects include negative effects on the central and peripheral nervous system (tremor, headache, insomnia, paraesthesias, uncoordinated movements, confusion, convulsions, vertigo); adverse metabolic effects (glucose intolerance, hyperkalaemia, hypomagnesaemia); gastrointestinal effects; and leucopoenia, thrombocytopenia and anaemia. Dose adjustments in these mild and moderate side effects must be evaluated on a case-by-case basis assessing the risks of serious side or toxic effects and acute rejection development.

An overall holistic approach must be implemented in the postoperative period and during the chronic phase. Patients must be reviewed not only for the assessment of rejection of the transplanted graft and the development of opportunistic infections but also in regard to the maintenance of homeostasis and proper function of organs and systems. Apart from the ordinary analytical workup during each postoperative control and clinic visit, a good anamnesis of all organs and systems should proceed.

The most common alterations include:

- Renal disturbances (increased creatinine clearance and renal failure)
- Hypertension
- Hyperglycaemia and diabetes
- Osteoporosis and hip necrosis
- Hyperlipidaemia
- Pneumonitis
- Mucosal ulceration
- Poor wound healing
- Malignancies

Patients may present, though, different types of postoperative complications and side effects depending on the immunosuppression regime. It is imperative that surgeons caring for VCA patients are well informed about the potential risks and side effects of such drugs and work within a multidisciplinary team.

Graft Failure

Failure of transplanted tissues and organs may occur as a result of a non-reversible surgical complication (thrombosis of the vascular pedicles not amenable for revascularisation), non-reversible grade IV acute rejection (necrotising rejection), invasive necrotising infection or immunosuppression problems (alterations or noncompliance with the protocol). Any explanting of transplanted tissues should proceed only after formal informed consent has been obtained, including its consequences and alternative options.

In theory, explanting a face allograft should return patients to their pre-transplant morbid condition. However, during transplantation the ablation of the deformed/destroyed anatomic units and other tissues can create a defect that may make impossible to return the patient to the same condition. Functional impairment may be worse than the premorbid condition, even though all plastic surgery techniques are employed to correct it. The aim of any face transplantation protocol is to return patients with graft failure to a situation that mimics or is identical to the pre-transplant condition. Multidisciplinary team support is necessary to help patients to go through this catastrophic complication, especially psychosocial services. All team members must bear in mind that the only solution to this complication, despite excellent and complex reconstructive plastic surgery interventions, is a new face transplantation.

Malignancies

Similarly to any other SOT recipient, face transplantation patients may develop tumour malignancies as a side effect of the immunosuppression. Among other malignancies (skin tumours, de novo neoplasms) patients should be screened on a regular basis for the development of EBV-induced lymphoma. It is a well-known complication of immunosuppression in transplant patients that deserve special attention. Specific treatment must be implemented to treat this disease. There are significant differences between SOT and VCA recipients. In the event of a non-responding patient or in patients with severe risks for side effects of the cancer treatment, it may be necessary to decrease or stop the immunosuppression to achieve a correct immunological response against the malignancy. During this treatment, patients may show acute rejection episodes and even graft failure. Therefore, full informed consent must be obtained before this protocol is started.

8.3   Appendix 8.1: Postoperative Orders

1. Diagnosis.
2. Check vital signs according to ICU protocol.
3. Check fluid balance every hour.
4. Tracheotomy care as per ICU protocol.
5. Central line management as per ICU protocol.

6. Nihil by mouth (exception, oral medications).
7. NG tube to gravity.
8. Urinary catheter and control of hourly urine output.
9. Check drains every 2 h.
10. Chest X-ray on admission to ICU.
11. Control of anastomosis with hand-held Doppler every hour for the first 24 h and then every 2 h for 6 days.
12. Blood test on admission to ICU:
    (a) Blood gas analysis with lactate and calcium (ion)
    (b) Complete blood cell count, platelets, prothrombin and partial thromboplastin ratios, fibrinogen, AST, ALT, bilirubin, GGTP, calcium/magnesium/phosphate, sodium/potassium/chlorine, total proteins, BUN, creatinine and glucose
13. Daily blood test:
    (a) Complete blood cell count, platelets, prothrombin and partial thromboplastin ratios, fibrinogen, AST, ALT, bilirubin, GGTP, calcium/magnesium/phosphate, sodium/potassium/chlorine, total proteins, albumin, BUN, creatinine, glucose and tacrolimus level
14. Cross-match on first day post transplant.
15. IV fluids as per protocol ICU and patient response.
16. IV broad-spectrum antibiotics according to institution guidelines (cover Gram+ cocci and Gram– bacteria):
    (a) Continue 3–5 days.
    (b) Change to appropriate antibiotics when surveillance microbiological results from donor and recipients are available (or PCRs).
17. Antifungal prophylaxis (liposome amphotericin 1 mg/kg IV).
18. Trimethoprim/sulfamethoxazole IV every 24 h until good oral tolerance; start then 80 mg PO 3 times per week.
19. Ganciclovir 5 mg/kg bid until good oral tolerance (if recipient– and donor+)
20. Tacrolimus 0.15 mg/kg/24 h IV in perfusion 24 h; switch to PO when good oral intake and correct IV levels
21. Thymoglobulin 2 mg/kg IV in IV perfusion (over 12 h). Premedicate patients 30 min before administration with prednisone 2 mg/kg, Benadryl 1 mg/kg, and acetaminophen 10 mg/kg.
22. Prednisone 2 mg/kg/day.
23. Topical tacrolimus 0.1 % 2 times per day for 2 months (start 10 days postoperative).
24. Mycostatin oral rinses every 8 h.
25. Omeprazole 40 mg/24 h.
26. AAS 100 mg PO every 24 h (3 weeks).
27. Low molecular heparin s.c. when platelet count >100,000.
28. Check capillary glucose every 6 h.
29. Insulin in sliding scale.
30. In case of rejection, start protocol (boluses of methylprednisolone) followed by daily quick taper:
    (a) First day, 5 mg/kg/day = _____ mg IV Q 6 h (divided in 4 doses)
    (b) Second day, 4 mg/kg/day = _____ mg IV Q 6 h (divided in 4 doses)
    (c) Third day, 3 mg/kg/day = _____ mg IV Q 6 h (divided in 4 doses)
    (d) Fourth day, 2 mg/kg/day = _____ mg IV Q 6 h (divided in 4 doses)
    (e) Fifth day, 2 mg/kg/day = _____ mg IV Q 12 h (divided in 2 doses); continued overtime mandated by clinical course

Infection Control

9

Abstract

As in any other transplant discipline, prevention of infection begins before the surgical intervention (the face transplantation). The most relevant issues during this phase are an adequate selection of donors and a complete workup in any recipient included in the face transplant programme. This evaluation is aimed to investigate and treat, if indicated and feasible, any infections present in recipients.

9.1 Infection Control Prevention

9.1.1 Pre-transplant Phase

As in any other transplant discipline, prevention of infection begins before the surgical intervention (the face transplantation). The most relevant issues during this phase are an adequate selection of donors and a complete workup in any recipient included in the face transplant programme. This evaluation is aimed to investigate and treat, if indicated and feasible, any infections present in recipients.

9.1.1.1 Donor Selection

Donor evaluation follows similar criteria and pathways as in the selection of donors for multiple-solid-organ donation. The transplant team addressed any general and formal legal issues and protocols in place for any given country. It is very important to remind that when the evaluation is performed in any immigrant donor, a very careful evaluation is mandatory, since there is the possibility to import certain exotic infectious diseases in recipients. Under this circumstance, any exotic viral and bacterial infections should be ruled out, and any vector for encephalitis discarded. When a donor becomes available and is considered for multiple organ donation, a full panel in blood test is run, including tissue typing, ABO and rhesus typing, serology for common infections and hepatitis, CMV and Epstein–Barr. Special attention must be paid in VCA donors to multiple resistant microorganisms; thus microbial culture of the nasal fossa and nasopharynx is mandatory. Current PCR tests provide results few hours after full evaluation.

9.1.1.2 Evaluation of Candidates

The transplant infectious disease specialist is a key team member of the transplant team. His/her full evaluation and recommendation before, during and after the transplant is extremely relevant to avoid significant complications and medication side effects during the whole lifespan of the transplant recipient.

Infectious disease specialists interview and evaluate patients during the whole initial evaluation of candidates and deliver their advice/prevention/treatments. During this evaluation, special attention is focused on current or past immunosuppression treatments, known allergies to antimicrobials and a thorough anamnesis of infectious diseases (Table 9.1). Apart from the past medical history regarding exposure to infectious disease vectors and diseases, the team focuses on other social issues such as travel to endemic locations for certain diseases (endemic parasitic and mycosis diseases), exposure to tuberculosis and past results of skin tests or chest X-ray alterations, risk factors for transmission of diseases in blood transfusions and current and future contact to children. Domestic issues are also explored. They include pets, nutritional habits (raw meat, seafood, no pasteurised milk and milk products, etc.) and type and origin of tap water.

A complete physical examination focuses on similar issues. It should uncover any current or past medical history/exposure to any microbial vector that may have implications in the transplant population. The physical examination is completed with a dental exploration and urological/gynaecological examinations.

Special explorations during this phase from an infectious disease perspective include tuberculosis

Table 9.1 Infectious disease anamnesis in VCA

Mouth: caries, sinusitis, pharyngitis, herpes virus infections

Respiratory tract: previous pneumonias, tuberculosis

Cardiovascular system: cardiac valve diseases

Gastrointestinal system: diverticulitis, diarrhoea, hepatitis (A, B or C), parasitic infections

Genitourinary system: urinary tract infections, prostatitis, vaginitis, genital herpetic diseases, other sexually transmitted diseases, condylomas

Skin: cutaneous or nail infections, varicella zoster

Osteoarticular: osteomyelitis, joint prosthesis

Childhood infections

Other infectious diseases: Epstein–Barr, HIV, *Brucella*, etc.

Previous exposures to infectious vectors

assay, chest X-ray and face sinus X-ray exploration. Face CT scan performed during the general face transplantation candidate evaluation should focus on active sinus disease and teeth exploration in order to rule out any active problems. They should be treated before the patient enters active search for donors. Multiple resistant bacteria deserve special attention. Patients that have had multiple hospital admissions and operations and stay in intensive care units are possible vectors for these bacteria. Nasal, pharyngeal and tracheotomy cultures are mandatory to explore the possibility for reservoirs.

Blood tests are drawn to check common serology of relevance for posttransplant immunosuppression; they include the following:
- Cytomegalovirus
- Varicella zoster
- Herpes simplex virus (1, 2, 6)
- Epstein–Barr virus
- Hepatitis panel (A, B, C)
- Human immunodeficiency virus (HIV)
- HTLVI, HTLVII
- Toxoplasmosis
- Syphilis

More than ever, in a global world, patients that are referred or have migrated from countries with known exotic infectious diseases must be explored for endemic infections that may develop during or after the transplant. They may include the following:
- Regional mycosis (histoplasmosis, coccidioidomycosis)
- Malaria
- Chagas disease
- Strongyloidiasis
- Amoebiasis
- Trypanosomiasis

Any positive finding should be individually investigated and treated if indicated. Patients that are reservoirs for multiple resistant bacteria are treated accordingly to eradicate the colonisation.

9.1.1.3 Vaccinations/Preventive Medicine

Preventive medicine professionals are important partners of the transplant infectious disease team. As in any other medical discipline,

Table 9.2 Current advice for vaccinations in face transplantation

Priority order	Type of vaccine	Pre-transplant	Posttranspant	Revaccine
1	Varicella	Last dose before 1 month to transplant	Contraindicated	
2	Rubella, parotiditis, measles			
3	Pneumococcus	Last dose before 2 weeks to transplant	Minimum 6 months after the transplant	1 dose at 5 years
4	Hib			
5	MCC			
6	Flu			Yearly
7	Hepatitis B			Depends on titres
8	Hepatitis A			1 dose if no response
9	dT			Every 10 years

the ideal scenario is to prevent any infections or disease in order to avoid complications and the necessity to start medications, treatments and hospital admissions. Infections and metabolic alterations may lead to rejection episodes, end organ failure and hospital readmissions and transplant failure. Table 9.2 lists the current vaccination protocol active in our institution.

Likewise to the psychosocial evaluation, infection control and preventive medicine focuses also on friends, social circle and family members of recipients. Physicians review and evaluate with the patient any person that will continue to have a close relationship; they may serve as vectors for viral and specific bacterial infections. Maintenance of a good immunisation in this close social environment is a must. Table 9.3 shows relevant vaccines in face transplant recipient contacts.

Table 9.3 Recommended vaccines in face transplant recipient's contacts

Vaccine	Recommendation
Parotiditis, rubella, measles	Close contacts (not in children under 12 months) and health personnel
Varicella	
Flu	Long-term contacts (more than 6 months) and health personnel. Annual vaccine
Hepatitis A	Long-term contacts (more than 12 months)

9.1.2 Transplant Day

During the active search for donors (active transplant waiting list), patients are followed at regular intervals to check health status and note any new events or the appearance of any symptoms. Transplant procedures require an intensive and aggressive induction of immunosuppression and long-term immunosuppression treatment. Patients are immediately at risk for developing bacterial and viral infections. As soon as there is a compatible donor, the patient is admitted to the hospital and a complete anamnesis and physical exploration follows to rule out any active infection. If the patient is CMV negative, serology is checked at this moment. The exploration is completed with a chest X-ray and tracheotomy and nasal swabs to determine the presence of any multiple resistant bacteria. Active acute infection contraindicates face transplantation at this moment.

Prophylactic antibiotics are administered to the donor during procurement. A broad-spectrum antibiotic active against gram-positive cocci and gram-negative bacteria (in special *Pseudomonas aeruginosa*) is indicated.

If microbiology results are available or any PCR is positive for specific bacteria, prophylactic antibiotics are adapted. It is mandatory to obtain blood for microbiology cultures and serum to run a complete serology test for common viral infections. During donor evaluation all these explorations are performed. However, patients are at risk for developing any serious bacterial and viral infections during the stay in the intensive care unit.

Face transplantation follows similar guidelines and protocols in recipients. The same type of antibiotic is utilised in the recipient unless specific isolates are present and known at this moment from the donor or recipient. Patients are immunosuppressed (they have received an intense immunosuppression induction) though; thus, antifungal drugs are administered during the transplantation to protect recipients against these types of infections.

9.1.3 Posttransplant Prophylaxis

Available literature on infection control and treatment in composite tissue transplantation is scarce. However, aside from immunosuppression complications, acute infections, especially during the postoperative period, are some of the most serious complications that a face transplantation patient may suffer in this stage. Table 9.4 lists the most important issues in posttransplant microbiological prophylaxis.

Antibiotic prophylaxis is commonly stopped between day 3 and 5 posttransplant. Special situations may force to prolong or change the administration of antibiotics. They include donor's positive blood culture (during procurement) and graft infection. Antibiotics should be adapted to the sensitivities and prolonged for a period of 10–15 days.

Antifungal prophylaxis is directed against *Candida* spp. and *Aspergillus* spp. Intravenous prophylaxis for *Candida* lasts for 3 days. Increased risks include patients that require dialysis, those who present with a creatinine

Table 9.4 Posttransplant prophylaxis tenets

Antibiotics (duration depending on donor's and recipient's results)
Antifungals (consider longer duration in intense immunosuppression)
Pneumocystis
CMV

clearance of less than 50 ml Kg/h or those who have more than 2 positive microbiology results (colonisation). In these situations, it is advised to prolong the treatment for a minimum of 15 days or as long as the risk is present. *Aspergillus* prophylaxis is performed with aerosolized antifungals, initially three times a week and then once a week. It is considered when the patient has received an intense immunosuppression: anti-lymphocyte serum antibodies or dialysis.

Composite tissue allotransplantation recipients commonly receive steroids as part of their immunosuppression regime. They are also the basis for the treatment of rejection episodes. They increase the risk for fungal infections and pneumocystis pneumonia. Prophylaxis treatment is based on the administration of co-trimoxazole for as long as the steroid therapy is continued. There are different oral presentations that allow for different treatment regimens. Some patients develop allergy or bone marrow toxicity. Leukocyte count has to be monitored during the acute phase (several medications have bone marrow toxicity). Nebulised pentamidine is an alternative in these situations.

Prevention of cytomegalovirus infection (CMV) is another pillar of infection prophylaxis in VCA. Prophylaxis is normally indicated in recipients that are CMV negative (never have had an infection of CMV) who receive an organ of a CMV-positive donor (the organ may serve as a vector for CMV and transmit the infection to the recipient; R−/D+). CMV infection in the immunocompromised host may be serious and life threatening; hence some VCA teams do not accept a CMV mismatch (R−/D+) to avoid serious complications. Moreover, it has been postulated that CMV replication may be a trigger for acute rejection. Prophylaxis is normally started with ganciclovir IV until it can be switched to valganciclovir PO. The treatment prophylaxis is continued until day 100 posttransplant and discontinued. Viral replication is monitored with real-time PCR or blood antigen levels at each clinic visit. Indications for treatment are listed *in* Table 9.5.

Table 9.5 Indications for CMV treatment during the first year posttransplant

1. Antigen blood levels >1/10^5 PMN·ml
2. >400 copies DNA/mL of blood
3. Acute rejection
4. Concurrent OKT3 treatment

Serum levels are necessary in children and in any patient receiving valganciclovir.

9.2   Treatment of Infections in VCA

Transplantation recipients are chronic patients that receive different type of medications that affect organs and systems and may produce important side effects. Some of the drug regimens present with potential side effects and toxicity. Antimicrobial therapy may produce adverse effects in transplant recipients; thus, a team approach is necessary to treat infectious complications in transplant recipients. Adverse effects may be produced by direct pharmacological interaction or by added toxic effect on organs.

9.2.1   Bacterial Infections

Empirical treatment should be started as soon as there is the clinical suspicion of a serious bacterial infection. We may differentiate graft infection and distant infections in other organs and/or systems. Infection of the face graft must be individualised. Each recipient receives different type of tissues and face structures, either intraoral, extraoral or both; the infection can be community or hospital acquired, and there may be deep abscesses. Treatment is normally dictated on a case-by-case basis; surgical debridement may be necessary in serious cases and in the presence of purulent collections. In severe cases or septic shock, empiric treatment should be initiated as soon as possible with broad-spectrum antibiotics (daptomycin and meropenem IV).

Other common bacterial infections in the transplant population include intraabdominal infections, pneumonia, IV-line sepsis and acute pyelonephritis. In all these situations, team members need to differentiate between hospital- and community-acquired infections and infections with high severity scores or sepsis. One should always refer to the current local or institution's treatment guidelines for specific treatment.

9.2.2   Viral Infections

The presence of any viral infection in a VCA patient may be the consequence of high levels/toxic levels of immunosuppression. This situation should always be explored and immunosuppression medications reduced if possible. The most common viruses encountered in VCA are herpes simplex, varicella zoster and CMV. Table 9.6 lists the most common herpes simplex and varicella-zoster infections. Oral treatment is indicated to limited and benign conditions (oral acyclovir, famciclovir, valacyclovir), whereas endovenous treatment is indicated in severe cases (acyclovir).

CMV infection is a common complication in the transplant population. Severe infections may trigger acute rejection episodes, have a significant impact in systems and organs and affect graft survival. Common infections in the transplant population are listed in Table 9.7. The decision-making process for VCA infection therapy is directed by viral load and the previous immunisation status of recipients. We must make a distinction between negative recipients (R−) and positive recipients (R+) who receive an organ from either a negative (D−) or a positive (D+) donor. In a mismatched recipient (D+/R−), all infections must be treated regardless of viral

Table 9.6 Common herpetic and varicella infections in transplant recipients

1. Herpes simplex:
Noncomplicated mucocutaneous infection
Severe mucocutaneous and visceral infection
Meningoencephalitis
2. Varicella zoster:
Localised in dermatome
Disseminated varicella-zoster infection

Table 9.7 Common CMV infections in VCA

Viral syndrome and hepatitis
Gastrointestinal disease
Pneumonitis

Table 9.8 Common *Candida* spp. infections in transplant recipients

Mucosal candidiasis
Oesophageal candidiasis
Candidemia
Peritonitis
Urinary infection
Asymptomatic candiduria

load. In all other cases (D+/R+ and D−/R+), current advice is to treat infections with a viral antigen load >25 or more than 2,500 copies in real-time PCR. Ganciclovir and valganciclovir are the treatment of choice. The response to treatment is monitored with viral antigen load in blood samples. Treatment should be continued until a negative viral antigen load is achieved in peripheral blood.

9.2.3 Fungal Infections

Candida and Aspergillus infections are the most common pathogens encountered in the transplant population (Table 9.8). Face VCA may include different amounts of mucosa, tongue, face bones and sinuses. Special attention must be directed to these areas to detect initial stages of mucosal mycosis. Mucormycosis may also develop in sinuses; hence X-ray examination and biopsies may be necessary in some circumstances. Treatment for *Candida* spp. depends on the stadium (initial, recurrent or therapeutic failure) and location. Initial phases are commonly treated orally with azoles (co-trimoxazole, fluconazole) or nystatin. Complicated cases, candidemia, peritonitis and fungal infections are treated intravenously (i.e. anidulafungin, amphotericin B) (Table 9.8).

Psychological and Psychiatric Evaluation

Abstract

The psychological and psychiatric evaluation of all candidates for face transplantation focuses on the identification of any risk factors that may have a direct impact in the development of postoperative complications or problems with self-adaptation and treatment compliance. Strong medical evidence demonstrates that the adaptation to posttransplant life, treatment adhesion and morbidity are directly related to specific psychosocial factors. In general terms, a detailed psychosocial evaluation of all patients is necessary before they are included in a transplant waiting list. Given the experimental nature of vascularised composite tissue allotransplantation, the psychosocial evaluation is mandatory. This is a formal requirement of the face transplant protocol and ethics committee. A negative psychosocial evaluation contraindicates VCA.

The psychological and psychiatric evaluation of all candidates for face transplantation focuses on the identification of any risk factors that may have a direct impact in the development of postoperative complications or problems with self-adaptation and treatment compliance. Strong medical evidence demonstrates that the adaptation to posttransplant life, treatment adhesion and morbidity are directly related to specific psychosocial factors. In general terms, a detailed psychosocial evaluation of all patients is necessary before they are included in a transplant waiting list. Given the experimental nature of vascularised composite tissue allotransplantation, the psychosocial evaluation is mandatory. This is a formal requirement of the face transplant proto- col and ethics committee. A negative psychosocial evaluation contraindicates VCA.

The evaluation and support by psychosocial services may be divided in three different stages:

I. Candidate for face transplantation
II. Immediate posttransplant period (up to 6 months posttransplant)
III. Chronic posttransplant period (6 months posttransplant onwards)

There are certain disease characteristics that the patient has to face and adapt to. Some patients will present with a disease that may be present from birth or may have appeared during growth; such is the case of benign neoplasms (neurofibromatosis) and vascular malformations. Others may have a traumatic aetiology; hence the patients had to

J.P. Barret, V. Tomasello, *Face Transplantation: Principles, Techniques and Artistry*,
DOI 10.1007/978-3-662-45444-2_10, © Springer-Verlag Berlin Heidelberg 2015

adapt to a sudden change in face appearance and quality of life. Patients included in the latter group present with special needs that differ from patients that had a prolonged period of adaptation to face disfigurement and change of quality of life. The motivation of the patient is crucial for the determination of a good indication for a face transplantation. The overall goal of face VCA is improvement of function and quality of life. Those patients that are well adapted may not benefit much from a face transplantation. Risks and side effects, hospital readmissions and change of life to a chronic condition (regular visit to clinic, biopsies and immunosuppression) are not uncommon, and the patients may not obtain a complete psychosocial improvement. Personal circumstances, social and family support, individual expectations and overall impact of the deformity need to be evaluated and explored to assess the potential benefit of the proposed treatment. The process does not only affect the postoperative adaptation to the new situation. Patients have to undergo a long evaluation process that includes hospital stay, procedures and techniques that may also induce psychological disadaptation, through an impact on their family, social and ethical environment. Psychological support has to be directed also to this initial phase. Some individuals may be well adapted to their situation before the possibility of a new treatment for improvement has arisen. During or following full evaluation, they can show high levels of anxiety and psychosocial problems. Therefore, the support has to be implemented and maintained for all patients, regardless of the final outcome of the candidacy evaluation.

The intervention of psychosocial health professionals, through a multidisciplinary approach within the face transplant team, is directed to:

(a) Allow the adaptation of patients to the process of evaluation and transplantation.
(b) Avoid or treat any psychological or psychiatric symptoms that may appear during the whole process.
(c) Provide continuous and permanent support to candidates and recipients and their families during the process of evaluation, search for donors and transplantation.

10.1 Candidate for Face Transplantation

10.1.1 The Evaluation Process

The overall goals during the evaluation phase include:

1. Detect the predictive risk factors that could interfere in the efficacy of the treatment.
2. Determine, through psychosocial exploration, the adaptation capacity and the patient's adhesion to the proposed treatment.

The psychological, psychiatric and social evaluation should focus in any past psychiatric history, drug or toxic abuse and any other factors that may prevent good confrontation with social and daily living events. The evaluation includes the three main spheres:

• Personality
• Social and family support
• Current quality of life

Common tests that are employed during the evaluation of the psychosocial status include the global psychiatric evaluation status (MINI), general humour and anxiety (HAD) and cognitive status (mini mental state exam [MMSE]). Table 10.1 lists common tests utilised in the psychological evaluation of transplant candidates.

During the different interviews with the psychosocial team, all levels of patient's interaction with his/her premorbid, morbid and projected post-morbid status are explored. A full history and exploration of the face deformity, family and personal psychiatric history and previous treatments, current psychiatric and psychological disorders and current treatment are explored and noted. It is very relevant to comprehend how the

Table 10.1 Common administered tests in transplant psychological evaluation

1. TCI-67-R: personality test
2. HAD: anxiety and depression
3. LOT: coping skills
4. DUKE: social support
5. SMAQ: compliance
6. SF-36: quality of life

patient understands, accepts and behaves in front of his/her deformity, not only in terms of his/her personal ability to cope with but also his/her interaction with family relationships and society in general. The family response to the current deformity and the response to other relatives' diseases have to be explored; they will signal how the family response and support could be expected after a face transplantation.

The patient is also questioned regarding the proposed treatment: fantasies about face transplantation, current expectations, level of knowledge of current scientific events and outcomes. An ambivalence attitude and curiosities and questions regarding the donor are also evaluated. The patient's sense of vulnerability is another issue of attention. Moral values and the way the patient copes with the current disease and any other previous health problems are important issues to determine his/her psychological status and determine future risks during the posttransplant period.

Another important component of this evaluation is the determination of patient's compliance with past visits, admissions and adhesion to treatments. It cannot be overstated that this is a very relevant issue. The success of any transplantation procedure is the compliance with medications, protocols, admissions, clinic visits and any other technique or procedure that may be necessary during the posttransplant period. Failure to take the medication regime and adhere to protocols may provoke transplant failure, side effects, infections, rejection episodes and death. The psychosocial team evaluates the relation of patients with their doctors and the compliance with any clinic visits, medications and diets. The former aids in the evaluation of the predisposition of patients to chronic treatments and the way they cope with anxiety and patience. Bad adherence to posttransplant treatments causes 21 % of all posttransplant complications, and it is the cause of 26 % of all posttransplant deaths (in the overall solid organ transplant series). Unexplained failure to attend clinic visits and bad communication of new symptoms are red flags of poor compliance. Another evidence is unjustified decreased level in serum of medications.

Table 10.2 General psychosocial indications for transplantation

Favourable psychiatric/psychological evaluation
Understand the face transplantation technique/treatment
Understand all obligations of face transplantation
Social stability
Absence of drug abuse during the last 2 years
Alcohol, benzodiazepines, cannabis abstinence of more than 6 months

The psychological and social factors that correlate with the abandon of treatment include:
1. Low educational level
2. Inappropriate social support
3. Marital status: single or divorced
4. Age below 40
5. Altered personality
6. Depression symptoms or anxiety in the post-transplant period
7. Bad communication skills
8. Opposition
9. Failure to recognise the disease process

The evaluation finalises with a complete exploration with all relevant tests of the current psychopathological symptoms, cognitive status and psychopathological diagnosis.

The final step of the psychosocial evaluation constitutes the development of the indication's document. This is a formal requirement during the whole evaluation process and relevant information for the Ethics Committee deliberation. As a matter of fact, there must exist an indication from the psychological and psychiatric standpoint in order to be able to proceed with the transplantation process. Some relative contraindication may be treated or a final decision postponed until more active fieldwork has been performed. General psychosocial indications and contraindications are listed in Tables 10.2 and 10.3.

During the psychological and psychiatric evaluation, social services are involved in order to explore the social support and the domestic situation of the candidate. The social network, type of relationships, close emotional relationships, economic status and type of home are fully evaluated. Any alteration that has occurred is deemed to have

Table 10.3 Psychosocial contraindications for solid organ transplantation (Strouse 1996)

Absolute contraindications:
Active drug abuse
Active mental illness/psychosis that limits significantly either:
Informed consent
Treatment adhesion
Active suicide ideation
Patient's absence for transplant consent
Factitious disease
Relative contraindications:
Inadequate social support
Dementia or permanent cerebral dysfunction in case of bad psychosocial support for good treatment adherence or progression to major neuropsychiatric disorder
Unable to cooperate with the transplant team; including psychiatric disorder with bad treatment response, humour alteration, schizophrenia, eating disorders and personality disorders

an impact on the patient and on the final outcome of any transplant. Some social situations provide full support for face VCA; others need some intervention before the transplant is ever indicated. The report of social services is included and evaluated in full by the psychosocial team to make a final report on the suitability of the candidate.

10.1.2   Patients on Active Waiting List

All recipients that have gone through the evaluation process and are considered candidates for face transplantation must be followed up and controlled by the psychosocial team for as long as the search for donors is active. Patients are followed up periodically at clinic visits with the psychologist, psychiatrist and social worker. Visits may be individual, joined by the family or in therapy groups that include family members and/or transplanted patients. The main goals of therapy groups include:

- Exchange of information. It will help patients to better understand the disease or deformity.
- Verbalising wrong feelings or cognitive errors regarding the operation and donors.
- Informing about the treatment, side effects and benefits of the face transplant.

Patients in the waiting list should have easy access to the psychosocial and the whole transplant team. It is not uncommon to follow a long period of time in the waiting list until a donor becomes available. Periods of stress and anxiety are not uncommon; they should be detected and treated promptly. The patient must be reinforced on a regular basis to maintain the positive expectations of the face transplantation.

10.2   Immediate Posttransplant Period (Less Than 6 Months)

This is an intensive period of particular relevance. The patient needs to adapt to his/her new appearance and a new reality that includes an intensive medical interaction, tests and procedures. Recipients learn their new situation, in particular new social relationships and their new medical environment: medications, tests, clinic visits, monitoring side effects and signs of rejection, etc. During the initial period, psychosocial intervention limits to adapt the patient to this new situation and modulate any alteration on the previous status.

In the months to follow, the psychosocial team focuses its attention to detect the appearance of mental and behaviour alterations of multifactorial aetiology: surgical interventions, anaesthetic effects, drug side effects, sensorial and personal isolation, intense re-elaboration of personal image, etc.

A special focus should be paid to relevant signs and symptoms that may interfere with a correct postoperative course and outcome:

- Acute and subacute episodes of confusion and dreamlike feelings
- Depression and depression symptoms
- Other humour alterations
- Cognitive alterations
- Sensorial and perception alterations

The treatment should be directed to make any preventive actions to avoid any psychological signs and symptoms that could affect the correct recovery and treatment adhesion. Other measurements are focused on psychopharmacological and psychotherapy treatments to modulate any psychosocial alterations during this phase of treatment.

10.3 Late Posttransplant Period (More Than 6 Months Posttransplant)

There is a significant difference between VCA recipients and any other solid organ recipients. Face VCA recipients have a significant change in their quality of life after face transplantation. Previous conditions do not affect directly health status. Patients are stable; their condition significantly affects quality of life but does not have an impact on organs and systems. There exist significant deformities, but in general terms, there is no need for any medical treatment. Patients may have been operated on several occasions, but this is a sole consequence of their deformity, not a question of disease. Life after VCA changes in many relevant levels. Quality of life is significantly improved in terms of social, family and work-related relationships. However, their health status changes to that of a chronic medical condition (not existing before the transplant). Patients are obliged to adhere to medical treatments, clinic visits, monitoring of rejection and side effects and hospital readmissions. Moreover, patients are normally in an excellent health status; thus long-term survival after the transplant is expected (all organs and systems have good physiological reserve to sustain medication side effects). The former makes multidisciplinary team follow-up mandatory. The psychosocial team must visit the patient regularly, most commonly during the same transplant team visit, when medications, rejections and health status not only are reviewed but also psychological well-being is monitored. All recipients should reach an excellent relationship with the psychosocial team and be provided with a direct line should any problem may arise.

Psychologists, psychiatrists and social workers favour active participation of recipients in individual and group interviews in order to achieve and maintain
- Independence
- Responsibility in treatment adhesion
- The rehabilitation process
- Social and work-related reintegration

The patient is the centre of the whole process, although special care is paid to involve the family and any carers. The whole process may have an important impact in both recipients and their families/carers. Hence any changes of alterations in the latter should be monitored and treated.

Immunological Aspects and Immunomodulation

Abstract

Vascularised composite tissue allotransplantation (VCA) is a new transplant discipline of reconstructive plastic surgery that relies on the restoration of deformity and/or amputation by the allotransplantation of different tissues and organs from another person (the donor). As in any other solid organ transplant discipline, graft survival depends on the acceptance of transplanted tissues and organs on the recipient and the absence or control of rejection episodes. In 1997, the Louisville team proved that long-term survival of transplanted limbs could be achieved in an experimental model with a triple-drug therapy (steroid, tacrolimus and mycophenolate mofetil). Soon afterwards, the first human hand transplants were a reality in 1998. The first experiences received the same immunosuppression regime, with excellent long-term results (both functional and immunological) to date. The current success of VCA is a promising field in plastic and reconstructive surgery. Intense research is currently being undertaken to improve the immune tolerance of composite tissues, since long-term results and face or limb acceptance depend on immune regulation and the control of side effects.

11.1 Introduction

Vascularised composite tissue allotransplantation (VCA) is a new transplant discipline of reconstructive plastic surgery that relies on the restoration of deformity and/or amputation by the allotransplantation of different tissues and organs from another person (the donor). As in any other solid organ transplant discipline, graft survival depends on the acceptance of transplanted tissues and organs on the recipient and the absence or control of rejection episodes. In 1997, the Louisville team proved that long-term survival of transplanted limbs could be achieved in an experimental model with a triple-drug therapy (steroid, tacrolimus and mycophenolate mofetil). Soon afterwards, the first human hand transplants were a reality in 1998. The first experiences received the same immunosuppression regime, with excellent long-term results (both functional and immunological) to date. The current success of VCA is a promising field in plastic and reconstructive surgery. Intense research is currently being undertaken to improve the immune tolerance of composite tissues, since long-term results and face or limb acceptance depend on immune regulation and the control of side effects.

J.P. Barret, V. Tomasello, *Face Transplantation: Principles, Techniques and Artistry*,
DOI 10.1007/978-3-662-45444-2_11, © Springer-Verlag Berlin Heidelberg 2015

Face VCA implies the transplantation of diverse tissues, such as skin, muscles, bones, lymph nodes, nerves, blood vessels, cartilage, soft tissues, salivary glands and mucosa. Given the nature of all these tissues, it is very difficult to parallel the immunological results of face VCA to that of solid organ transplantation. Face VCA is composed of different tissues with diverse types of immunogenicity and immune response. There is some consensus on the general type of immunosuppression regime that is necessary in VCA, although the perfect drug combination is still to be defined. However, functional outcome depends much on tissue survival and the immunological response; thus immunomodulation during induction, immediate postoperative period and long-term follow-up is very relevant for the final outcome and the improvement in quality of life.

11.2 Immunological Aspects of VCA Tissues

11.2.1 Skin

The cutaneous component of face VCA is an important part of the face graft. It is what we see, how we feel, the interaction with society and the basis for expression. Its colour, quality, structure and texture indicate to others our emotions, age, temper and health.

The skin is a highly immunogenic tissue with active immunological functions. Apart from the structural layers (epidermis and dermis), the skin has resident cellular elements and cells in transit with immunological and pro-inflammatory properties. This particular immunological microenvironment is termed skin-associated lymphoid tissues (SALT). Cells that participate in this system are diverse (Table 11.1); the most important part of it includes antigen-presenting cells (APC). This microenvironment is responsible to drain to the regional lymph nodes and report its status. It is very relevant in transplant physiology for up and down immunological regulation and for the development of short- and long-term tolerance.

Table 11.1 Skin-associated lymphoid tissues (SALT)

1. Antigen-presenting cells (APCs):
Langerhans cells
Dendritic cells
2. Lymphocytes
3. Keratinocytes
4. Fibroblasts
5. Endothelial cells
6. Local/regional lymph nodes

The functions of cutaneous antigen-presenting cells include:

• Expression of high levels of class I and II antigens of the major histocompatibility complex (MHC)
• Expression of CD80 and CD86 (molecules for co-stimulation)
• Internalisation and process of antigens
• High capacity of migration (allows for antigen transportation)
• Stimulation of allogenic T cells

Cutaneous APCs (Langerhans cells and dendritic cells) are normally inactive in a stationary status; however, a few numbers of cells migrate to regional lymph nodes to present antigens on a regular basis, which allows for a status of tolerance. Under certain circumstances (i.e. inflammatory stimulus), APCs respond in an intense manner; this response allows for a correct reaction against the insult, whereas the slow-rate migration maintains the tolerance against self antigens.

Other immunological skin resident cells include T cells, which are normally present within the dermis. They are represented by CD4 cells (T-helper subpopulation) and CD8 (T-suppressor and cytotoxic). T-helper cells may be subdivided into Th1, memory cells responsible for the initiation of the cell-mediated response (they secrete pro-inflammatory cytokines IL-2, IL-12 and IFN-γ) and Th2 (they produce IL-4, IL-5, IL-6, IL-10 and IL-13) responsible for B-cell response.

The immunological response can also be started by keratinocytes. They are a source of pro-inflammatory cytokines IL-1, IL-6, IL-8 and TNF-α; they have a systemic effect on the immune system, modulate the proliferation of keratinocytes and attract inflammatory cells. IL-7 and IL-15 contribute to the circulation of T cells; and IL-10, IL-12 and IL-18 are responsible for the systemic response. The stimulation of keratinocytes with IFN-g produces the expression of MHC class II proteins and intracellular adhesion molecule I (ICAM-I), which explains that keratinocytes play a role both as APC and in the induction of functional immune reaction.

11.2.2   Regional Lymph Nodes

Transplantation of composite tissues carries with it a certain amount of lymphatic tissue, mainly in the regional drainage lymph nodes and in the bone marrow should the VCA include bone. Nodes are a source of immunocompetent T cells, B cells and follicular dendritic cells. They contribute to the immunological response of the transplant on the recipient. Competent recipient's T cells migrate to the regional lymph node of the transplant and they proliferate. When immunosuppression drug levels are inadequate, they may trigger an acute rejection episode. On the other hand, cutaneous dendritic cells may migrate into the regional lymph node and trigger a secondary immunological response when in contact with the recipient's T cells.

11.2.3   Muscle

Face transplantation is intended not only as a restorative operation but also a quality improvement therapy. Face muscles play an important role in quality improvement, especially face sphincters (oral and orbital), which restore important functions. An absent inflammatory and immune response in the muscular layer is necessary to maintain a good functional outcome. Under physiological conditions, muscle cells do not express MHC class I or II molecules (they do express class II molecules in in vitro culture of muscles cells stimulated with IFN-a, IFN-g and IL-1b). Hence, we may hypothesise that muscle cells may express class II molecules in certain viral and bacterial infections, present antigens

and produce autoantigens. On the other hand, skeletal muscle expresses HLA-G, a MHC class I molecule that is involved in immune tolerance.

11.2.4   Peripheral Nerves

Correct reinnervation of the transplanted face is responsible for an adequate sensation and motor function of face muscles. Peripheral nerves include different cell types and tissues: neuronal axons, Schwann cells and connective tissue. Connective tissues and cellular elements of the immune system are present in the epineurium and perineurium. Schwann cells may produce different pro-inflammatory cytokines (IL-1, IL-6, TNF-α), other mediators (prostaglandin E, thromboxane A, leukotriene C) and immune modulators (TGF-β). Schwann cells express MHC class I antigens in normal circumstances. Following nerve injury, they express class II antigens and IFN-g in the presence of activated T cells. This suggests that Schwann cells may function as APC (antigen-presenting cells) and play a role in local immune response. Immunomodulation is mediated through the production of erythropoietin. It prevents axonal degeneration, reduces the production of TNF-α, prevents Wallerian degeneration and diminishes neuropathic pain. Transient activated T cells and B cells can be located in peripheral nerves, independently from antigen specificity. APCs are normally represented by local macrophages, expressing MHC class II antigens and co-stimulating molecules B7-1 and B7-2, which are essential in T cells for antigen presentation and local immune response.

11.2.5   Bone and Bone Marrow

Face bones are an integral part of face transplantation when the mandible and/or the maxilla are reconstructed. Immune bone antigenicity is considered to be low. However, limb and face VCA may include bone marrow, which carries with it a significant amount of haematolymphoid cells. In adequate conditions, the transplantation of bone marrow cells in non-myeloablative immunosuppression creates a status of immunomodulation and downregulation of the recipient's immune system and can be involved in the induction of tolerance. Following limb or face VCA that includes bone marrow (or in research protocols for tolerance induction with infusion of donor's bone marrow), haematopoietic and donor's lymph cells migrate (including dendritic cells and APCs) from transplant tissues and colonise lymphoid and non-lymphoid recipient's organs (chimerism). When these migrating cells colonise and react against the recipient's tissues, graft-versus-host disease may develop, which may be fatal.

11.2.6 Blood Vessels

Face transplantation follows the same principles of reconstructive microsurgery. In general terms, the face graft can be conceived as a free flap prefabricated by nature and harvested from another human being. Correct circulation with enough inflow and adequate outflow is necessary for flap survival. Endothelial cells play a multifactorial function: regulation of haemostasis, cell adhesion, vasomotor tone regulation and immune regulation. The latter is mediated by leucocyte and other immune cells' adhesion and migration across the endothelium. In inflammatory conditions, endothelial cells produce IL-1, IL-6 and IL-8 and activate the expression of P selectin, E selectin and cellular adhesion molecules (ICAM-1, ICAM-2 and VCAM-1), which facilitate leucocyte migration. They also facilitate the proliferation and differentiation of activated T cells and Th memory cells through APC, MHC class II molecules and CD40 co-stimulating molecule.

11.2.7 Salivary Glands and Oral Mucosa

Salivary gland immune function is mediated through the mucosal cells and the associated lymphoid system. Acinar and ductal cells excrete glycoproteins for IgA and IgM. Lymphoid sys-tem is located in a diffuse manner within the glands and in regional lymph nodes. This tissue is an important effector site for the immune reactions of the oral mucosa and regulates the cellular and antibody immune reactions. Flow cytometry differentiates mononuclear cells of T, B and NK origin.

Oral mucosa is an integral part of most face transplants. Its physiologic function includes the recognition and elimination of pathogens and tolerance of commensal bacteria necessary for immune homeostasis. The most important cells of mucosal immune reactions are dendritic cells. They express CD1a molecules for the presentation, activation and maturation. Other identified cells in oral mucosa include dermal and plasmacytoid dendritic cells which contribute to the pool of CD83+ dendritic cells of the basal lamina and to viral antigen presentation. Other immune elements of oral mucosa include lymphoid and myeloid cells, such as basal lamina cells, dendritic cells and CD4+ T cells with expression of CD45RA and CD45RO.

11.3   Immunological Monitoring

11.3.1 Pre-transplant Evaluation

The monitoring and immunological outcome of face transplants depend on risk factors that should be evaluated in the overall candidate evaluation such as the determination of donor-specific preformed antibodies (DSA). During the overall evaluation in the pre-transplant phase, tissue typing (HLA), anti-HLA screening and compatibility tests are performed. The experience in other solid organ transplantation indicates that high levels of DSA should be avoided to reduce the risk of hyperacute rejection.

HLA typing has been traditionally performed by serological methodology. However, recent work indicates that most laboratories are currently utilising molecular tests for tissue typing, including primer-specific PCR sequencing (sequence-specific primer [SSP]), specific sequencing of oligonucleotide primer (SSOP) and direct DNA sequencing. Typification of donor and receptor HLA allows:

- Evaluation of correspondence in HLA
- Excluding donors with HLA antigens in recipient's preformed DSA

HLA matching is not a formal requirement in face transplantation. The paucity of donors would make face transplantation almost impossible, although the real implication of mismatching is still to be evaluated. Renal transplantation literature indicates that HLA-DRB1 matching is a priority. In general terms HLA or tissue typing is essential in transplantation medicine. Good compatibility shall indicate a correct or optimal outcome, whereas a low match or complete mismatch may increase the rejection episodes in VCA recipients. In renal transplantation, the better the tissue compatibility, the longer the renal graft functions and survives in the long term. Previous transfusions, transplants and pregnancies may increase the risk for sensitisation and production of donor-specific antibodies and HLA antibodies. Cross tests between donor's and recipient's lymphocytes depict the lymphotoxicity in the presence of complement. A positive cross-match test shows the presence of antibodies in the recipient's serum against class I molecules and should be considered a contraindication for transplantation.

11.3.2 Posttransplant Monitoring

The main objective of posttransplant control and monitoring is to make an early detection of acute and/or chronic rejection and side effects of immunosuppression protocols. It does include anamnesis, clinical inspection, complete physical examination, laboratory tests and skin/mucosa biopsies:

1. HLA monitoring

    This type of monitoring is very relevant to determine the potential for acute and chronic graft injury. There exists strong evidence that the presence of donor-specific antibodies highly correlates with acute and chronic rejection. It is mandatory to monitor antibodies for HLA-A, −B, −Cw, −DR and −DQ

donor antigens, since they predict graft failure.

2. Non-HLA antibodies

    They may be both allo- and autoantibodies. They also signal tissue injury and the possibility for chronic and progressive graft failure, although they are not as specific as anti-HLA immunoglobulins. They correlate to non-HLA antigens of the major histocompatibility complex class I coded in A chain (MICA), other endothelial antigens, minor histocompatibility antigens, vascular receptors, adhesion molecules and intermediate filaments.

3. T-cell function

    T-cell subpopulations are closely monitored during the immediate posttransplant period (following induction therapy) in order to check for an adequate immunosuppression and profound deletion of lymphoid cells. They are then checked at regular intervals to assess the efficacy of immunosuppression drugs and avoid over-immunosuppression.

4. Transplant tolerance

    This is a field of intense research in solid organ and VCA allotransplantation. One of the main focuses of novel immunomodulation therapies is the induction and maintenance of antigen-specific tolerance. It is defined as the maintenance of a functional graft with long-term survival in the absence of active immunosuppression. Achieving long-term tolerance in the clinical scenario of VCA is extremely difficult given the complex heterogenicity of composite tissues and the donor–recipient immune environment. There have been clinical experiences of immune tolerance induction through mechanisms of downregulation and immune anergy with minimal or no immunosuppression. The former may be produced by partial clonal deletion, clonal anergy, changing the cytokine expression panel and the stimulation of immunoregulatory cells. In general terms, one should consider the status of immune tolerance as a temporal or permanent downregulation status regardless of the mechanism of action according to Sachs. In many clinical situations, it is achieved by means of the maintenance of minimal non-toxic doses of immunosuppressive drugs, which may be completely irrelevant. Calne has termed this manoeuvre a status of "quasi-tolerance", aiming for long-term survival of a functioning transplanted organ and absence of acute or chronic rejection, significantly reducing the side effects of immunosuppression therapies. A similar type of action of tolerance with minimal immunosuppression has been proposed by the stimulation of immunoregulatory cells. Tolerance development may be obtained in peripheral lymphoid tissues (peripheral tolerance) or centrally through a thymus mechanism of action. Other proposed experimental methods for tolerance induction in VCA include donor's bone marrow infusion, monoclonal antibodies and the stimulation of gamma–delta T cells.

5. Anamnesis, clinical inspection and laboratory tests

Daily inspection and search for signs and symptoms of rejections is necessary immediately posttransplant and thereafter for the rest of the life. Both patients and clinicians should monitor possible side effects and medication toxicity. Signs and symptoms for systemic hypertension, infections, hypercholesterolaemia, lung toxicity, skeletal abnormalities and renal failure must be included. Patients are carefully reviewed at each visit and a complete laboratory analysis is performed. They should include haematological markers, general biochemistry, lipid metabolism, lymphocyte subpopulations, hepatic and renal function, viral real-time PCR in the first year posttransplant and drug serum levels. Overall clinical impression and laboratory tests mandate immunosuppression dug adjustment if needed.

During the immediate postoperative period, graft vascularisation is monitored with direct periodical clinical inspection and hand-held echo Doppler.

Duplex-Doppler or angio-computed tomography (CT) scans are helpful to diagnose any flow alterations. During this phase and for the rest of the postoperative period, the graft is closely monitored for signs of acute rejection. The patient is subsequently trained to perform his/her own daily inspection and to detect any early signs and symptoms of acute rejection.

There does not exist a biochemical marker for acute or chronic rejection in VCA. Therefore, rejection is controlled by clinical inspection and tissue biopsies when indicated by the daily evaluation.

Immunological monitoring includes:
– Inspection of the transplanted graft
– Skin and muscle biopsies as mandated by clinical inspection
– Serum levels of immunosuppression drugs
– Study of lymphocyte subpopulations

6. Tissue biopsies

The absence of biochemical markers (such as those encountered in hepatic and renal transplantation) makes tissue biopsies (skin and mucosal biopsies) necessary for the confirmation of suspected acute rejections. It must be noted that these biopsies should be taken into consideration together with the clinical picture. The presence of perivascular mononuclear infiltrations or any other alteration in keratinocytes or tissue structures is not a sole indication for acute rejection. Pathological findings should be evaluated with the clinical inspection and sign and symptoms to reach a formal diagnosis. On the other hand, clinical signs of rejection must be confirmed by tissue biopsy. In the absence of pathological confirmation, other causes for clinical findings should be investigated.

Histopathological signs for acute rejection include:
• Mononuclear infiltration of skin, mucosa or both
• Immunoglobulin or complement deposition
• Oedema
• Cellular necrosis
• Intimal hyperplasia
• Fibrosis

Indiscriminate utilisation of tissue biopsies should be avoided. They may compromise the final aesthetic result of the face graft (multiple

Table 11.2 UHVH skin/mucosal biopsy protocol

1. Biopsy on day 0:
   Donor's biopsy pre-procurement
   Biopsy after revascularisation
2. Biopsy on day 7
3. Biopsy on day 14
4. Biopsy on day 30
5. Biopsy every month during first year posttransplant
6. Ad hoc biopsies in case of clinical signs and symptoms of rejection

Table 11.3 Banff classification of composite tissue allotransplantation rejection

Grade 0	Nonspecific changes
	No or only mild lymphocytic infiltration without involvement of the superficial dermal structures or epidermis
Grade I (mild rejection)	Superficial perivascular inflammation with involvement of superficial vessels and without involvement of overlying epidermis
Grade II (moderate rejection)	Features of grade I with involvement of the epithelium and adnexal structures
Grade III (severe rejection)	Band-like superficial dermal infiltrates with more continuous involvement of the epidermis and middle and deep perivascular infiltrates
Grade IV (necrotising rejection)	Features of grade III along with frank necrosis of the epidermis and other tissues

scars). Transplanting extra tissue in the neck or lateral area of the transplant and the utilisation of a sentinel flap are approaches that different teams have proposed to minimise the impact of multiple skin biopsies on the final outcome of the face allograft transplantation. However, gravity and congestion in the cervical region may alter some results by deposition of cells in this area. Sentinel flaps, on the other hand, may show also different results than those observed in the face transplantation (the tissue characteristics may differ). Signs of rejection in one location and absence of such episode in another have been observed; hence results should be carefully evaluated. Our current protocol for skin/mucosal biopsies is depicted in Table 11.2.

During the Banff meeting in A Coruña, Spain (Banff CTA-07), experts reached a consensus for the grading of pathological tissue rejection in VCA, incorporating classifications grading the severity of acute rejection (Table 11.3). Tissue biopsies should be obtained from a specimen of a minimal diameter of 4 mm including skin, dermal annexes, dermis, subcutaneous tissues and blood vessels. In case of a suspected acute rejection, biopsies should be obtained from erythematous indurated cutaneous areas. Recommended laboratory process includes haematoxylin and eosin (H&E) and periodic acid–Schiff (PAS). Depending on results and other experimental protocols, immunohistochemistry assays may include (but not limited) CD3, CD4, CD19, CD20, CD68, HLA-DR, CMV and C4d.20 and immunoglobulin deposition. Unless the clinical situation mandates otherwise (necrotising rejection, ulcers, severe functional impairment), the treatment for acute rejection is halted

until a definitive diagnosis is obtained. In contrast to other solid organ transplantation, functional impairment does not affect vital functions; thus definitive treatment can be temporised. On the other hand, intense over-immunosuppression may alter or have a significant impact on other organs and systems and produce toxic levels or chronic side effects.

11.4 Immunosuppression in Face Transplantation: The Clinical Experience

Few reports in medical literature are currently available for the immunosuppression in composite tissue allotransplantation, mainly from clinical experience in the first cases of face transplantation and the cumulative experience in hand transplantation. More relevant information may also be obtained from the international registry on hand and composite tissue allotransplantation (IRHCTT), which can be accessed online at the international registry website.

In general terms, all protocols base the immunomodulation of VCA on an induction therapy with lymphocyte-depleting agents and a triple-drug therapy of tacrolimus, mycophenolate mofetil and steroids (prednisone or methylprednisolone). Acute rejection episodes are normally steroid sensitive. In some cases lymphocyte-depleting agents are utilised with a tapering of high doses of steroids; others use boluses of steroids with a quick taper. Chronic immunosuppression is based mainly on three-drug therapy, although changes from calcineurin inhibitors to sirolimus or other drugs, steroid-sparing therapies and others have been implemented in some cases. Current experience indicated that the induction therapy with lymphocyte-depleting agents may induce a cross-reaction with up- and downregulation of allo-T cells. The activation and regulation of both auto- and allo-lymphocytes after transplantation and induction therapy may influence and promote peripheral graft tolerance.

The utilisation of different immunosuppressive drugs affects different immunological pathways with distinct infectious disease implications. The involvement of infectious disease specialists is mandatory to couple immunosuppression with the specific infection prophylaxis.

Table 11.4 Types of immunosuppressive agents

Pharmacological agents	1. Corticosteroids: i.e. hydrocortisone, methylprednisolone, dexamethasone
	2. Calcineurin inhibitors (CNIS): inhibitors of cytokine production; tacrolimus (Tac), cyclosporine (CsA)
	3. Antiproliferative agents: Inhibitors of cell cycle: mycophenolic acid (MPA), mycophenolate mofetil (MMF), azathioprine (AZA) mTOR inhibitors: rapamycin (RAPA) and everolimus (RAD)
Biological agents	1. Monoclonal antibodies: Anti-CD3 (OKT3) Anti-CD20 (rituximab) Anti-CD52 (alemtuzumab) Anti-CD25 Anti-IL-2 (basiliximab and daclizumab)
	2. Polyclonal antibodies anti-lymphocyte: Antithymocytic globulin from rabbits (r-ATG) Equine anti-lymphocyte globulin (ATGAM)

11.5 General Overview of Immunosuppressive Treatments

Correct and efficacious induction and maintenance of immunosuppression is crucial for excellent outcome, longevity of grafts and overall survival. Moreover, tapering drugs to achieve the minimal dose–effect ratio is important to avoid or minimise side effects and complications.

Current immunosuppressive drugs that are currently available for clinical use can be classified either as pharmacological or biological agents (Table 11.4). Other new agents include molecules that co-stimulate inhibitor proteins currently in research studies in autoimmune diseases and solid organ transplantation. All listed agents and drugs may be used during the induction therapy and maintenance therapy and for the treatment of acute rejection. Patients receive multiple pharmacological therapies for infection prophylaxis, intensive care support, treatment of other concomitant diseases and side effects or other conditions. These drugs may be introduced in the long term to treat any new medical problem related or non-related to the face transplantation. Physicians should be well trained in immunosuppressive treatment and maintenance in order to avoid interactions between medications that may alter the efficacy or blood levels of immunosuppressive agents.

11.5.1 Immunosuppressive Therapy

The main objective of immunosuppressive treatments includes maintenance of correct graft function, absence of acute and chronic rejection, achieving graft tolerance and the avoidance or minimisation of potential toxic or side effects of medications.

Strategies for the modulation of the immune response in transplantation medicine can be divided into two main phases or stages: the induction and the maintenance immunosuppression.

1. Induction therapy:

    The objective of the initial phase is to achieve an intense immunosuppression during the first week posttransplant in order to reduce the probability of early acute rejection. In general terms, induction therapy is performed by the intravenous infusion of a monoclonal or polyclonal antibody, which tends to reduce the severity of any rejection episode and favours the development of long-term tolerance. During this induction period, maintenance therapy is started and monitored to adjust the doses of drugs to the serum target and the clinical response.

2. Maintenance therapy:

    The scope of this immunosuppression protocol consists of a strategy to suppress the recipient's immunological response against the allograft, inhibiting their ability to recognise the foreign tissues and to organise an orchestrated response. The drug regimen is adapted on an individual basis to reach the minimal doses of medications that allows for a correct immunomodulation with minimal toxicity. Immune adaptation allows for decreasing doses of medications over time while maintaining the same effect. A treatment regimen that employs multiple drugs produces a synergistic and adjunctive effect of immunosuppression minimising toxicities.

3. Acute rejection therapy:

    First line of acute rejection therapy in VCA consists in high doses of glucocorticoids (they are normally steroid sensitive) and an optimisation of the immunosuppression regime. In some cases, though, monoclonal or polyclonal antibodies may be necessary when no responses or a partial response is obtained with intravenous boluses of corticoids. When the rejection episode is limited to the skin, topical steroids or topical tacrolimus creams may be indicated. Extracorporeal phototherapy has also been proposed to diminish sensitisation in selected cases. The treatment of acute rejection episodes requires the utilisation of high doses of medications that affect the immune system

and have profound implications in infection control and side effects. Severe acute rejections require hospital admission and prompt treatment.

11.5.2 Dose Adjustment for Side Effects

Immunosuppressive therapy is not risk free. Aside from the increased risk for infections, each agent can produce different adverse effects, which may be strengthened by other concomitant medications (Table 11.5). Mild to moderate side effects include negative effects on the central and peripheral nervous system (tremor, headache, insomnia, paraesthesias, uncoordinated movements, confusion, convulsions and vertigo), adverse metabolic effects (glucose intolerance, hyperkalaemia and hypomagnesaemia), gastrointestinal effects and leucopenia, thrombocytopenia and anaemia. Dose adjustments in these mild and moderate side effects

Table 11.5 Side effects of immunosuppressive agents

Agent	Key adverse effects
Cyclosporine	Nephrotoxicity, neurotoxicity, hyperglycaemia, hyperlipidaemia, gingival hyperplasia, hirsutism, hypertension, malignancy
Tacrolimus	Nephrotoxicity, neurotoxicity, hyperglycaemia, gastrointestinal disturbances, hypertension, malignancy, alopecia
Corticosteroids	Hypertension, hyperglycaemia, osteoporosis, growth retardation, cataract, gastrointestinal ulceration, poor wound healing
Azathioprine	Myelosuppression, hepatotoxicity
Mycophenolic acid	Myelosuppression, gastrointestinal disturbances, malignancy
Sirolimus	Hyperlipidaemia, thrombocytopenia, anaemia, poor wound healing, pneumonitis, mucosal ulceration
Anti-lymphocyte Ab	Cytokine release phenomenon, viral activation, immune complex syndrome

must be evaluated on a case-by-case basis assessing the risks of serious side or toxic effects and acute rejection development.

11.6   Immunology of Acute Rejection

Composite tissue allotransplantation grafts may be rejected through a cellular-mediated or humoral-based response of recipient's immune system against membrane antigens of donor's cells. The most potent antigens to promote this immune response are group A antigens of the human leucocyte antigen (HLA) system and AB0 antigens of red blood cells. It is possible to check beforehand or after the transplant the functional status of the immune system in vitro, thus typifying tissues and tissue compatibility.

The principal mechanism for allograft rejection (host-versus-graft reaction, HVGR) is the lymphocyte immune reaction (cellular-mediated) against the antigens of donor's tissues. HVGR is a retarded hyper-sensibility reaction (very similar to that of tuberculosis skin test). This reaction causes the destruction of grafted tissues in few days, and it is characterised by a mononuclear infiltrate with different degrees of haemorrhage and oedema. Vascular network seems to be spared, although the endothelial cells are also primary targets for this immune reaction. This immune cell-mediated rejection may be controlled by the intensification of immunosuppression; the areas that have been injured by the rejection episode heal with fibrosis, whereas the rest of the transplanted tissue has a normal appearance. If acute rejections are controlled and long-term survival of the grafted tissues is achieved, good long-term outcomes can be observed even with low doses of immunosuppression medications. This long-term adaptation/tolerance is probably mediated by the loss of highly immunogenic leucocytes (including dendritic cells) and the appearance of a donor-specific suppressive immunological response in the recipient.

Chronic rejection often develops in solid organ transplantation. It is seldom observed in VCA, although the longest follow-up comprises the initial experience in hand transplantation (up to 16 years). This type of rejection develops in an insidious manner and progresses regardless of immunosuppression levels. The true effector mechanism is still unknown, although current research indicates that a humoral response mediated by systemic antibodies may be relevant. The pathological picture differs from that observed in acute rejection. Endothelial damage and intima proliferation, which commonly progresses to complete vessel lumen obliteration, is observed. It gradually occludes vessels, causing tissue ischaemia and fibrosis of the transplanted organ. The role of a humoral response (systemic antibodies) is evident when the recipient has been sensitised against donor's antigens (pregnancies, blood transfusions, previous transplantations). If these preformed antibodies do exist, they commonly lead to a hyperacute rejection episode with complete organ destruction few minutes after transplant revascularisation. It is characterised by thrombosis of small-calibre blood vessels and micro- or macro-infarcts in the transplanted tissue (regardless of the type and intensity of immunosuppression induction). Similar responses are observed if a noncompatible AB0 group organ is transplanted to the recipient. There currently does not exist any immunosuppression that can control or treat these types of hyperacute rejections.

11.7   Appendix 11.1: HUVH Immunosuppression Protocol

11.7.1   Induction Therapy

1. Preoperative infusion of Thymoglobulin (atg) as soon as the patient arrives at the hospital, at a dose of 2 mg/kg. Premedicate with 1 g of methylprednisolone IV, Benadryl 50 mg IV and acetaminophen 650 mg PO.
2. Revascularisation: Administer 1 g of methylprednisolone IV, 30 min before revascularisation.
3. Thymoglobulin (atg), 2 mg/kg/day for 5 days (start preoperatively).

4. Methylprednisolone:
   - Days 1–14: Administer a dose of 2 mg/kg/day.
   - Taper down the dose of methylprednisolone over time to 10 mg/day.
5. Tacrolimus 0.15 mg/kg/day divided into two doses. Start treatment preoperatively.
6. Mycophenolate mofetil: Initial dose of 1 g two times a day (total dose of 2 g). Start preoperatively. Adjust according to leucocyte count and stop 1 year after the transplant.

11.7.2 Maintenance Therapy

1. Tacrolimus: Serum target levels of 10–15 ng/ml during the first 6 months (months 1–6 posttransplant) and target levels of 5–10 ng/ml after 6 months posttransplant.
2. Mycophenolate mofetil: Adjust levels according to leucocyte count.

3. Methylprednisolone: Taper down levels to 10 mg/day. Consider lower levels or alternate levels if good response.
4. Topical tacrolimus 0.1 % 2 times/day for 2 months (start on day 10 posttransplant).

11.7.3 Treatment of Acute Rejection

1. Increase the dose of tacrolimus if serum blood level is <15 ng/ml.
2. Methylprednisolone, 1 g/day/IV for 3 days.
3. If severe rejection: Methylprednisolone 5 mg/kg IV in 4 doses with quick taper over 5 days.
4. Consider topical tacrolimus and steroids.
5. Steroid-resistant rejection:
   (a) OKT3 5 mg/day/IV for 7 days
   (b) Thymoglobulin (atg) 2 mg/kg/day for 3 days
6. In repeated severe acute rejections, consider extracorporeal photopheresis.

Specific Aspects of Anaesthesiology in Face Transplantation

12

Abstract

Face transplantation is a novel experimental treatment that aims to reconstruct face deformity by the replacement of face anatomy with donor tissues. However, the anaesthetic act does not differ much from common surgical interventions in plastic and reconstructive surgery. In general terms, massive bleeding (burns, head and neck tumours, neurofibromatosis, etc.) is common to some operations, and autotransplantation (free flaps, microsurgery) is performed on a daily basis.

Face transplantation is a novel experimental treatment that aims to reconstruct face deformity by the replacement of face anatomy with donor tissues. However, the anaesthetic act does not differ much from common surgical interventions in plastic and reconstructive surgery. In general terms, massive bleeding (burns, head and neck tumours, neurofibromatosis, etc.) is common to some operations, and autotransplantation (free flaps, microsurgery) is performed on a daily basis.

Preoperative and intraoperative anaesthetic management and postoperative care of face transplant patient mandate a thorough knowledge of plastic surgery techniques and transplantation medicine. Face transplantation should only be contemplated in tertiary university hospitals that have a tradition in transplantation and can provide assistance of all clinical and basic services anytime during the entire year. A multidisciplinary approach should be contemplated, which warrants a robust team discipline and good control and prompt treatment of side effects and possible complications. The implication of the anaesthesiology department and the development of a thorough anaesthetic protocol are necessary for excellent outcomes.

12.1 Preoperative Assessment

It is part of the general evaluation of candidates and it allows risk assessment and planning of the operation and preparation for individual necessities. A general consensus does exist among all transplant disciplines, transplant coordination and the transplant unit in order to proceed with multiple-heart-beating-organ donation that suits different surgical specialities. Anaesthesiology assessment is an integral part of the candidate's evaluation; the overall risk, his/her classification in one of the ASA

J.P. Barret, V. Tomasello, *Face Transplantation: Principles, Techniques and Artistry*,
DOI 10.1007/978-3-662-45444-2_12, © Springer-Verlag Berlin Heidelberg 2015

system and the indication or contraindication from an anaesthetic perspective are a part of the decision-making process in an indication for face VCA. The implication of an anaesthesiologist well experienced in both transplant surgery and plastic surgery microvascular free flap surgery is essential for the success of the procedure, and we highly advice this approach.

Preoperative assessment includes a broad anamnesis, history of the face deformity (causes and consequences), co-morbidities and a battery of preoperative tests/explorations.

12.1.1 The Face Deformity

Airway assessment is a must. Patients that require a face transplantation to reconstruct the face deformity are expected to have an important alteration of normal anatomy. The maintenance of a patent airway before, during and after the surgical intervention is crucial to achieve an uncomplicated hospital course and good tissue oxygenation and pulmonary function. Some patients will have a permanent tracheotomy as part of their deformity. It is recommended that it be maintained until the VCA has been performed and a correct airway has been achieved after the transplantation. For the rest of the patients, the risk for an oral intubation is evaluated. If orotracheal intubation is feasible, it will be carried out and converted to a tracheotomy after induction. Some other patients may have a high risk for orotracheal intubation. In this population, it is advised to perform a tracheotomy under local anaesthetics and sedation.

12.1.2 Cardiac Assessment

A complete 12-lead electrocardiogram and chest X-ray are obtained. Past medical history regarding operations, arrhythmia, exercise tolerance and stress response is explored. Other special explorations, depending on past medical history and other findings, may include echocardiogram and treadmill exercise.

12.1.3 Central Line Evaluation

During face VCA an important amount of blood loss may occur. Good venous access with large calibre lines is essential for correct and prompt fluid replacement (Fig. 12.1a, b). During the physical examination, common sites for central line insertion are inspected. It is recommended to obtain a minimum of 2 accesses, one multiple-line central line access for the administration of medications and fluid and one large-bore access for fluid replacement.

12.1.4 Lung Function Evaluation

It follows the same tenets of cardiac evaluation. A broad anamnesis and physical exploration are first, together with a chest X-ray. Next, depending on findings and past medical history, function tests, exercise tolerance and CT scan may be necessary to assess the overall function of the pulmonary system. Any pathological finding or alteration should be treated and corrected before the operation.

12.1.5 Renal Function

The response of the renal function during past operations is evaluated. History of past and current medications and their effect in kidney function is checked and noted. Important analytical studies include creatinine, urea, blood and urinary osmolality, potassium, chlorine, calcium, phosphate and magnesium.

12.1.6 Hepatic Evaluation

In general terms, an analytical evaluation of hepatic function suffices. It includes ALT, AST, GGT, bilirubin, alkaline phosphatase, albumin and total protein count. Past medical history that involves hepatic function alteration, glucose intolerance or hypoglycaemia during the stress response should be investigated.

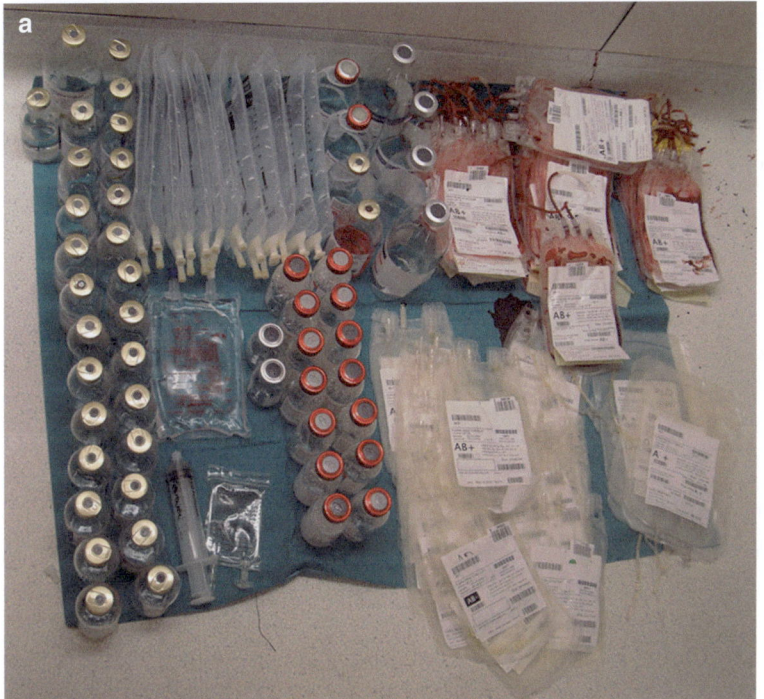

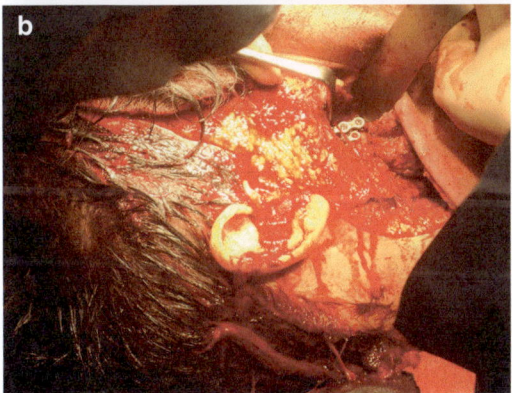

Fig. 12.1 (**a**, **b**) Massive blood loss may occur during VCA surgical operations. Good calibre central line access is essential for the success of the operation

12.1.7 Haematological Evaluation

A correct and successful outcome of any operation depends on a good oxygen delivery and correct red cell count to prevent any major unexpected haemorrhage. Good cardiac function is essential for a good cardiac output and oxygen delivery. Still, good tissue oxygenation depends also on a correct haemoglobin level.

General analytical workup includes haemoglobin, haematocrit and platelet count, prothrombin time, TTPA and fibrinogen. Patients that had previous bleeding complication or unexplained thrombosis or coagulation alterations require a special coagulation study. The haematological study is finished by a serology test for hep B and C, HIV, herpes viruses, CMV and Epstein–Barr.

12.2   Anaesthesia in Face VCA

12.2.1   Preoperative Orders

As soon as the patient arrives to the hospital, an urgent preoperative evaluation is carried out as in any other urgent plastic surgery patient and transplant recipient candidate. The preoperative anamnesis is discussed with the patient and any new medical event noted. An urgent blood test is obtained, including haematology, coagulation parameters and general biochemistry. The evaluation is completed with a chest X-ray and an electrocardiogram. A blood sample is also obtained for cross-match; a total of 10 units of packed red cells and 10 units of fresh frozen plasma are ordered. The operation should not start until the packed red cells and plasma are not physically in theatre (similarly to major burn wound surgery).

12.2.2   Anaesthetic Preparation

An important part of safe surgery protocols is a complete preoperative checklist. The anaesthesiologist must check the following together with the anaesthetist nurse:

1. Monitors, ventilator, material and theatre (Table 12.1)
2. Medications (Table 12.2)
3. Emergency set (Table 12.3)
4. Haemodynamic medications (Table 12.4)
5. Antibiotic prophylaxis
6. Immunosuppression

Material for difficult airway manoeuvres, tracheotomy and cricotomy sets, different types of lines, IV access, etc. should be present in the operating room. A ventilator with positive end-expiratory pressure (PEEP) mode that may work in both volume and pressure modes is advised. It must be noted that all sets of medications, emergency medications, etc. should be adapted to every institution's standards. In general terms, the VCA theatre must be prepared as a high-risk procedure similarly to open-heart or complicated major burn surgery.

Table 12.1 Common checklist in anaesthetic preparation

Ventilator (volume/pressure modes)
Desflurane vaporiser
Capnography and pulse oximeter
ECG monitor
PICCO monitor
BIS monitor
4 infusion pumps (minimum)
Invasive arterial pressure and cardiac pressure modules
Echograph for central line placement
2 Hotlines (minimum)
Rapid infusion line set
Foleys
NG tubes
Core temperature probes

Table 12.2 Common medication list

1. Anaesthetic induction
Midazolam
Propofol
Atropine
Atracurium
Succinylcholine
Fentanil
2. Continuous perfusion pumps
Atracurium
Fentanil

Table 12.3 Emergency set

Atropine
Calcium chloride
Adrenaline
Lidocaine
Calcium bicarbonate
Furosemide

Table 12.4 Haemodynamic drugs

Noradrenaline
Dopamine
Dobutamine

Antibiotic prophylaxis is delivered according to the transplant protocol and the first dose started before the surgical incision as usual guidelines for clean surgery. Immunosuppression induction therapy is another feature of this initial anaesthetic

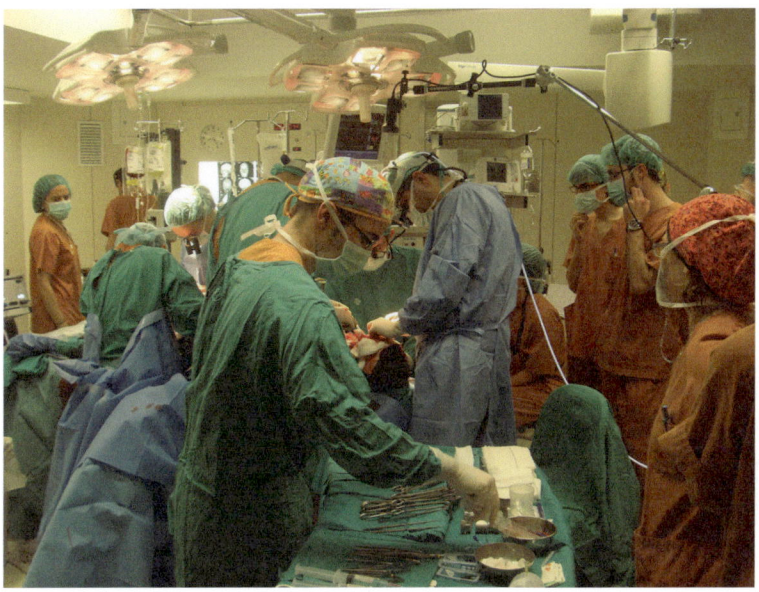

Fig. 12.2 Large and spacious operating rooms are necessary for correct VCA procedure management

phase. It is infused preoperatively, either after admission in the ITU room or in the operating room under strict control and monitoring. One gram of prednisone IV is advised 30 min before revascularisation. Ischaemia reperfusion of transplanted grafts may release an acute source of inflammatory cytokines; the whole transplant team must be aware of this issue and be prepared for a profound systemic response with a hypodynamic phase and shock.

12.2.3   Intraoperative Monitoring

There are two main stages that should be differentiated and that reflect the complexity of each phase. The first phase includes the induction of the anaesthesia, and it does not differ much from other plastic surgery operation. Monitoring is based on ECG monitor, non-invasive blood pressure and pulse oximeter. After anaesthetic induction and airway control, the maintenance anaesthetic phase is monitored through ECG monitor, pulse oximeter, capnography, direct blood pressure monitoring, pulmonary artery pressure, pulmonary capillary pressure, central venous pressure and extravascular lung water.

The monitoring is completed with BIS (level of sedation), urinary output (Foley) and core temperature monitoring.

12.2.4   Anaesthetic Management

Large operating rooms (50 or more square metres) that allow for good circulation of personnel and correct placement of all necessary material are advised to attempt face VCA (Fig. 12.2). It is not uncommon to join together during certain parts of the operation many surgeons, scrub nurses and anaesthesiologist, operating microscopes, hotlines and different operating side tables and other monitors that are normally in use during face VCA thus, enough space is necessary for a good outcome.

Patients are normally premedicated with midazolam, and an induction with a quick sequence is utilised, which prevents and avoids bronchial aspiration (it should be remembered that transplantation procedures are nonelective operations, and patients are not fasting). Anaesthetic maintenance is performed with desflurane, fentanil and atracurium or cisatracurium. Fluid replacement is advised by mixing normal saline and Ringer's lactate; blood replacement is dictated by clinical and laboratory response. During the operation, apart from continuous monitor control of vital signs, patients are routinely assessed every hour and before and after allograft revascularisation with specific laboratory and clinical signs (Table 12.5). Fluid balance is monitored with insensible fluid losses, operating field fluid/blood loss, urine output and overall blood loss, which are continuously assessed; special attention is paid during important bleeding phases of the operation and before the end of the operation.

Table 12.5 Hourly intraoperative control

1. Biochemistry:

   Check sodium, potassium, chlorine, calcium (ion), magnesium, lactic acid and blood gas analysis, glucose, urea, creatinine, total protein count and albumin

2. Haematology:

   Haematocrit and Haemoglobin

3. Coagulation:

   Prothrombin time, INR, TTPA, fibrinogen and platelets

4. Haemodynamics:

   Mean arterial pressure, pulmonary artery pressure, pulmonary capillary pressure, cardiac index, CC, heart rate

5. $EtCO_2$, FiO_2, SpO_2

6. Urinary output

7. Core temperature

Face Graft Procurement

13

Abstract

Face transplantation consists in the extirpation of face tissues of a donor with the diagnosis of brain death (solid organ donor) and its transplantation to a patient to reconstruct his/her face defect. All deformed and scarred recipient face tissues are removed and replaced by normal tissues, which restore anatomy and function.

Face transplantation consists in the extirpation of face tissues of a donor with the diagnosis of brain death (solid organ donor) and its transplantation to a patient to reconstruct his/her face defect. All deformed and scarred recipient face tissues are removed and replaced by normal tissues, which restore anatomy and function.

The main difference between classical microvascular autologous reconstruction and vascularised composite tissue allotransplantation relies on the procurement of the required tissues for reconstruction from a donor and the mandatory immunosuppression. Face tissues are obtained following allotransplantation concepts. It may incorporate an important quantity of composite tissues with arteries and veins that support the vascularisation of the transplanted face, similarly to that observed in autologous transplantation. The overall process follows similar tenets of autologous microsurgery utilised in reconstructive surgery. However, the participation of two patients in the whole process (the donor and the recipient) makes necessary the participation of two surgical teams and two operating rooms.

The donation of face tissues follows the same directives of solid organ donation. Donors shall be haemodynamically stable, although there is no contraindication for the use of vasopressors (the face is a highly vascularised organ). Donor relatives shall be informed of the tissues that are to be procured and they must provide informed consent for such donation (Appendix 13.1). Inclusion criteria for face donors are very selective because it has to be individualised for each recipient. In general terms, these criteria include:

1. Multiorgan donor with confirmed diagnosis of brain death
2. Signed informed consent from relatives for face donation
3. Compatibility of gender, skin tone, age, ABO blood group and rhesus and morphometrics

Exclusion criteria are very selective. They follow the same protocol existing for solid organ donation, although certain specific criteria are included (Table 13.1)

J.P. Barret, V. Tomasello, *Face Transplantation: Principles, Techniques and Artistry*,
DOI 10.1007/978-3-662-45444-2_13, © Springer-Verlag Berlin Heidelberg 2015

Table 13.1 Exclusion criteria for face donation

1. Sepsis and septic shock
2. HIV
3. Hepatitis B and/or C (with the exception of hepatitis B/C recipients)
4. Viral encephalitis
5. Cancer
6. Active IV drug abuse
7. Tattoos in the last 6 months
8. Inherited peripheral neuropathies
9. Inflammatory of infectious neuropathies
10. Systemic infections with associated neuropathies
11. Toxic neuropathies
12. Neurological neoplasms
13. Rheumatoid arthritis
14. Autoimmune diseases
15. Diseases of the collagen
16. Acute face trauma
17. Severe face deformity
18. Face paralysis

Table 13.2 Face VCA preoperative protocol

Blood test	Complete blood count, coagulation tests, general biochemistry, liver function tests, total proteins, calcium
Inform infectious disease specialist	On arrival
CMV and EPV serology	If CMV-/EPV-
Blood typing and cross-matching	Reserve minimum of 10 packed red blood cells, 10 units of FFP and 3 units of platelets
PRA	Not necessary if performed <3 months
Tissue typing	All patients
Antibiotics	According to institution's protocols
Chest X-ray	On arrival
Blood, urine, pharynx, tracheotomy microbiology cultures	On arrival before surgery
Inform and consult anaesthesiology	On arrival
Induction immunosuppression	Prepare and infuse induction medication according to institutional protocol (see Table 13.3)
If PRA >50 %	IV immunoglobulin complex G 2 g/kg

As soon as a donor has been identified and the recipient is confirmed (there may be more than one possible recipient in active search), the following steps must be performed:

- Confirm donation and recipient match.
- Activate preoperative protocol (Table 13.2).
- Call infectious diseases department to rule out any active infection.
- Obtain IV lines.
- Prepare operating room and all necessary equipment.
- Alert VCA multidisciplinary team.
- Start immunosuppression induction protocol (Table 13.3).

In general terms, face VCA procedures utilise a two-team technique approach—donor's and recipient's teams—similarly to that employed in SOT, especially in heart and lung allotransplantation (these two organs are very sensitive to ischaemia, and two-team approaches are normally implemented, where they work simultaneously to shorten the overall transplantation time).

As soon as a donor has been confirmed, the recipient is informed and he/she is admitted to the hospital. All preparations for surgery are then started. At the same time, the team in charge for

Table 13.3 HUVH induction immunosuppression protocol

If VCA is imminent with positive donor, start induction protocol with a minimum of 2 h before transplantation:

1. Thymoglobulin (ATG) 2 mg/kg on slow infusion rate
2. Premedicate 30 min before infusion with:
   (a) Prednisone 1 g IV
   (b) Diphenhydramine (Benadryl®) 50 mg IV
   (c) Acetaminophen 650 mg IV

face procurement is dispatched in order to obtain the face VCA. Tissue requirement varies, depending on the defect to reconstruct (partial or full face transplant), and so does the approach for the surgical procurement and the technique utilised during donation. However, regardless of the type of donation and technique utilised for the procurement, the fabrication of a face prosthesis must precede any VCA procedure (limbs, face,

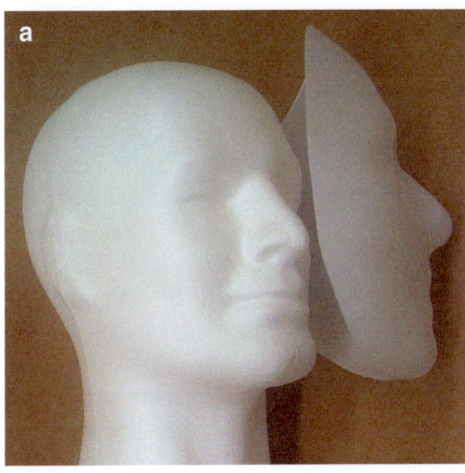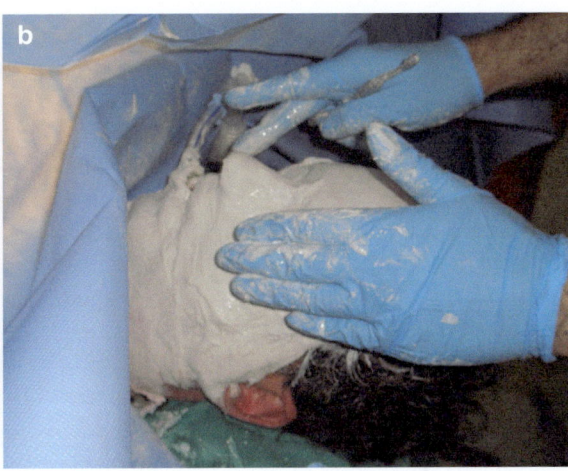

Fig. 13.1 (**a, b**) Face mask impression is necessary to maintain bioethics during face transplantation. It is best obtained in the ITU before the donor is transported to the operating room

etc.). Maintaining the dignity of the patient during the whole donation process is mandatory, and bioethics during procurement call for excellency in the care of the donor.

It is recommended to obtain an impression of the face in the intensive care unit well before the patient is transported to the operating room (Fig. 13.1a, b). Alternatively, the impression can be obtained before the donor operation, although logistics may be more cumbersome in this scenario (timing, space, surgical teams' pressure). Obtaining the face impression in the ICU has other positive points. It allows obtaining the impression unhurried and provides plenty of time for the prosthetics to manufacture a silicone or resin-like mask ready to use at the end of the procurement. The overall goal is not to produce a replica of the donor's face, but to provide dignity and an aesthetic closure of the face remnants. Relatives shall be informed that a close coffin funeral will be necessary, regardless of the perfection of the face prosthetic mask provided for the donor's reconstruction.

Another important issue in the logistics and the strategy for face VCA procurement is the type and timing of the operation. In general terms, similarly to many other face VCA teams, we recommend a heart-beating donation. It shortens the ischaemia time, reduces the impact of ischaemia–reperfusion injury and allows for correct haemostasis during the face procurement operation. However, other teams have implemented a non-heart-beating procurement (at the end of the multiorgan procurement), although experience has shown that it may produce a massive haemorrhage at the time of reperfusion and will prolong ischaemia time.

If the VCA team contemplates a heart-beating donation, good collaboration among all multidisciplinary team members and the rest of SOT teams is necessary. A multiple-organ donation in a heart-beating donor can be organised with two different approaches:

1. Face VCA procurement at the beginning of the operation (before all other organs have been procured—nonsynchronous procurement)
2. Simultaneous procurement of the face and internal organs (synchronous procurement)

13.1   Nonsynchronous Procurement

Under this strategy, face VCA procurement is performed at the beginning of the operation. Plastic surgeons obtain the face allograft in a similar manner to that executed in reconstructive flap procurement in autologous composite microvascular flap surgery. Face VCA retrieval is given priority and the rest of the teams wait for completion of the plastic part of the donation. At the end of the face VCA procurement operation, the face is perfused in a side table with cold (4 °C) preservation fluid, and it is transported to the recipient's operating theatre. Closure of the defect is performed in the usual manner by means of the application of a face prosthesis. The rest of the multiple-organ donation is then carried out. This approach has the convenience of an unhurried, relaxed face procurement, although it poses a significant risk for the rest of the internal organs and raises significant ethical questions. In fact, internal organ (lungs, heart, and liver) donation is intended to save lives, and as such it is the belief of transplantation medicine that it should be given priority. It is not uncommon to experience important blood loss and haemodynamic instability during face procurement, which could lead to cardiac arrest.

13.2 Synchronous Procurement

This is our technique of choice and it is our ordinary approach for VCA procurement. During our first face VCA (world's first full face transplantation), we proved this technique to be safe, feasible and effective. We believe that this technique follows bioethics guidelines and preserves the whole philosophy of transplantation medicine. Table 13.4 summarises the more important issues of this synchronous procurement.

Table 13.4 Main steps in synchronous face VCA procurement

Heart-beating donation
Consider tracheotomy
Preparation of face mask (consider fabrication in ITU)
Transplant teams evaluate internal organs
Catheterisation of major vessels *without* infusion
Face CTA procured in situ without osteotomies synchronous with in situ procurement of internal organs; face procurement halted
Preservation fluid infusion
Heart–lungs procured
Face (osteotomies), liver, pancreas, kidneys procured simultaneously with running cold preservation fluid
End of extraction

The operation begins securing a patent and safe airway. When face graft procurement is scheduled during a multiple-organ donation in a heart-beating donor, securing a patent and safe airway during face graft procurement is a must. Approaching the different anatomical parts that need to be dissected in order to obtain a total or partial face allograft requires several changes in head orientation. During each of these manoeuvres, airway decannulation or even accidental extubation may occur. In the event of such accidental extubation, the donor may arrest and challenge the whole organ donation. Tracheostomy may be performed in the ITU (surgical or percutaneous) or as a first step of multiple-organ procurement. A high incision is advised (first rings below cricoid cartilage) to allow for a long tracheal segment in case double-lung transplantation is planned.

If a face impression for a prosthetic mask has not been obtained in the ITU, it is then obtained and fabricated before all surgical teams start the procurement. It is advised to obtain it in the ITU, in order to speed up the process and prevent operating room contamination (Fig. 13.1).

The first step during multiple-organ donation including face VCA procurement is a median laparotomy and thoracotomy. The multivisceral transplant surgeons and cardiothoracic transplant surgeon evaluate the organs. If organs are valid, the recipient's operations elsewhere are started (ischaemia time tolerance for heart and lungs is low). Major vessels are cannulated in the usual manner and the procurement is halted. Cannulation of major vessels may be performed as follows:

(a) Cannulation of common carotid artery and internal jugular vein in the lower third of the neck (commonly used if there is no lung–heart procurement).

(b) Cannulation of aortic arch including the heart cannulation. The distal portion is clamped during preservation fluid infusion to force fluid into the cervical vessels. This is our preference when heart–lung procurement is planned.

Following major vessel cannulation (without infusion), in situ dissection may proceed. All

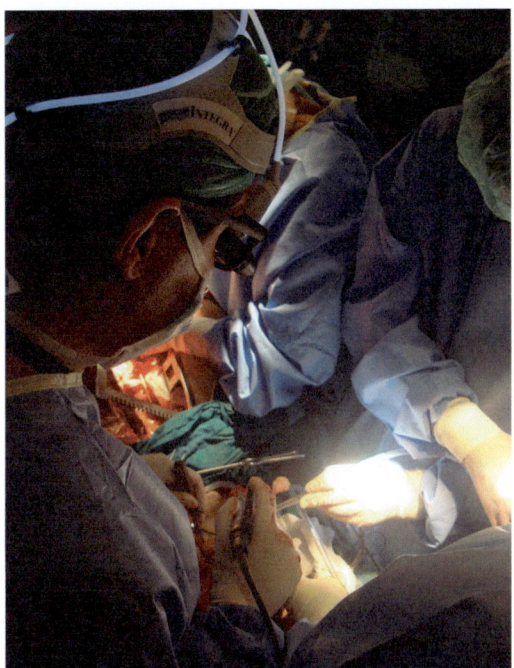

Fig. 13.2 Simultaneous in situ dissection of internal organs and face grafts required excellent organisation of teams in order to work in confined spaces. Experience surgeons should be included in the multidisciplinary team to expedite the operation. Note that thoracic/abdominal and face VCA teams work in close vicinity

infusion stations should be ready and all teams in stand-by should any instability or arrest forced immediate perfusion.

Synchronous in situ dissection is the next step (Fig. 13.2). Abdominal surgeons and plastic surgeons work together simultaneously to dissect and prepare the organs for the final step (infusion and final procurement). Ideally, this dissection is carried out until all necessary steps of surgical preparation have been performed. In the case of face VCA procurement, dissection shall be carried out until all attachments to the bony skeleton have been severed and the face graft is pedicled on major vessels. The second option involves halting the dissection at the time of osteotomies to avoid major haemorrhage from internal maxillary arteries. However, common carotid arteries may be clamped to avoid this complication.

When all internal and face grafts have been dissected, the operation reaches its final step.

Cardioplegic and preservation fluids at 4 °C are perfused and the donor is rapidly cooled. Major vessels are sectioned and all organs are ready for transportation. The organisation of the OR and the position of infusion stations are depicted in Fig. 13.3.

In the event of haemodynamic instability or cardiac arrest, the dissection is stopped and the infusion starts regardless of the status of the operation. Final steps of dissection are performed under running preservation fluid to allow for haemostasis or with extensive bank surgery before transportation.

Face grafts are then packed in the usual manner and dispatched to the recipient's operating room.

13.3   Human Resources in Face VCA Transplantation Procurement

An experienced team is necessary to perform a rapid and safe procurement that does not interfere with the rest of the donation process and allows for an efficient and correct organisation of face graft procurement. Experienced plastic surgeons with good knowledge of flap reconstructive surgery and craniofacial expertise should be included in the procurement team. Similarly, anaesthesiologists should be well versed in plastic surgery procedures and in those procedures that present with major haemorrhage and instability, such as major burn surgery and craniofacial surgery. In addition, we would recommend to include in the team a senior multivisceral transplant surgeon who shall help and assist during the whole process of donation, act as a leader and director for all transplant teams (shall assist in timing for cannula placement, dissection, infusion, etc.) and take care of liver procurement.

The organisation of human resources differs, though, and depends on the type of procurement:
1. *Nonsynchronous*: Face graft procurement is obtained in a non-heart-beating donor. Anaesthesiologist support is no longer necessary, and the team should be organised internally

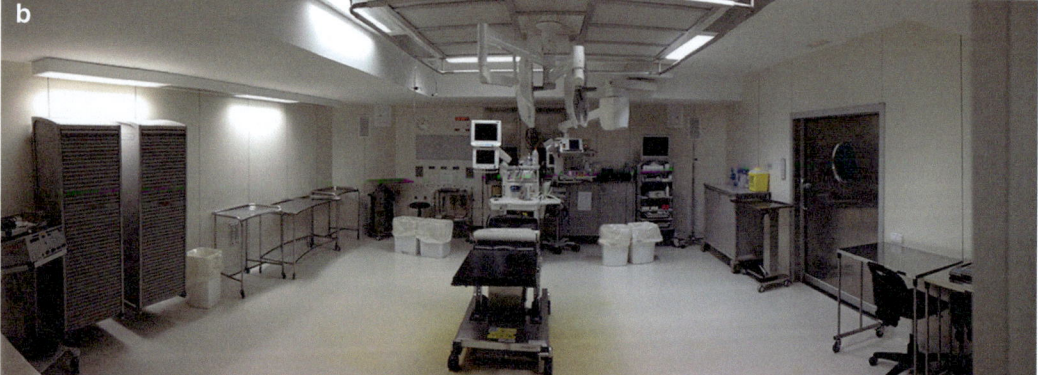

a

Anaesthesia station

Infusion pump

Abdomen

Feet

Thoracic scrub table

Operating table

Abdominal scrub table

Infusion pump

Heart

Head

Face VCA scrub table

Infusion pump

VCA-Face

b

Fig. 13.3 Organisation of infusion pump stations, surgical tables and anaesthesiologist station during synchronous multiple-organ donation including face VCA

within the plastic surgery department. In general terms, the team shall include three to four plastic surgeons (including residents in training), one scrub nurse, one circulating nurse and one transplant coordinator. The operation is performed under running preservation fluid, and it is advised that one transplant nurse remains in the operating room to take care of the pump and the rest of the transplant requirement (normally shared with renal surgeons).

2. *Synchronous*: A heart-beating multiple-organ donation including face VCA is one of the most complex surgical scenarios. Besides the usual human resources that are necessary to perform a classical multiple-organ donation, synchronous procurement of a face VCA graft requires the addition of specific personnel. One extra anaesthesiologist that is experienced in craniofacial surgery and difficult airway is necessary. This anaesthesiologist assists and helps the transplant anaesthesiologist to maintain patient stability and patent airway. One to two scrub nurses are necessary. The final number of nurses depends on the length of the operation, although the team should be prepared for a long surgical intervention. The plastic surgery table is normally situated at one side of the head of the patient, preferably on the right side. Three plastic surgeons (normally two faculty members and one senior resident) are necessary to perform face graft procurement in a safe and efficient manner. In normal circumstances, and extra plastic surgeon will be available for replacement of assistance in long or complex operations. The team includes also one circulating nurse, one transplant nurse that shall take care of the infusion pump station and one transplant coordinator.

13.4 Surgical Technique

The following is a general summary of face graft procurement. It may apply for different situations and institutions. Although it may differ in some technical points when we consider a heart-beating vs. a non-heart-beating donor procurement, the technique is explained as a whole.

13.4.1 Table Position and Airway Management

On arrival to the operating room, the operating table should be positioned in a standard craniofacial procedure (anaesthesia station at the feet of the patient), allowing for a complete freedom of movements around the patient. Extension tubing for airway management should be employed as needed. Both arms are best positioned parallel to the trunk. Again, extension lines should be used as needed.

If a tracheotomy has not been performed in the ITU, it is performed at this moment and airway is properly secured. Surgeons must remember to place a high tracheotomy incision to allow for a long tracheal segment in preparation for double-lung transplantation. Similarly, if a prosthetic mask impression has not been obtained previously, it is performed at this moment before the whole surgical intervention begins.

13.4.2 First Stage: Evaluation of Internal Organs and Cannulation

The patient is then prepped and draped in the standard fashion. The surgical area includes a wide area extending from the hypogastria and both inguinal areas to the thorax, neck and face in a single operative field. It is recommended that the face transplant instrument table is placed at the right side of the patient's head, whereas all instrument tables for thoracic surgeons and abdominal surgeons are placed at the left side of the patient, in order to allow for good circulation of personnel and allow good exposure for surgeons.

The operation starts with a standard abdominal incision and a median sternotomy in continuity. The type of incision is the surgeon's choice. As soon as haemostasis is achieved and good exposure of solid organs is obtained, the multivisceral and cardiothoracic surgeons evaluate the internal organs. If the organs are considered valid, transplant surgeons cannulate the major abdominal and thoracic vessels and leave the cannulas in situ. The infusion pumps are connected and the operation is halted at this stage. No infusion is started at this moment. During cannulation, the thoracic cannulas may be inserted in the aortic arch to allow for simultaneous infusion of the heart/lungs and face. An alternative to thoracic cannulation is common carotid cannulation above the clavicles.

In the event of an abdominal solid organ donation without heart/lungs procurement, the operation follows similar tenets with the exception of a median sternotomy. If this is the situation, the cannulation for face graft infusion is performed in the neck through the common carotid arteries.

13.4.3 Second Stage: Solid Organs and Face Graft In Situ Dissection

During this stage the dissection of the face graft begins. It is performed with simultaneous in situ dissection of solid organs; in special liver, pancreas and kidneys; and any intervention that may be appropriate in the thoracic organs. All transplant teams should stay in stand-by but ready for activation in case there is a sudden instability/arrest of the donor that mandate immediate infusion and preservation of organs. In our experience, this simultaneous in situ dissection is safe and feasible. Good organisation of teams is necessary since there is no extra room for all transplant teams (Fig. 13.4).

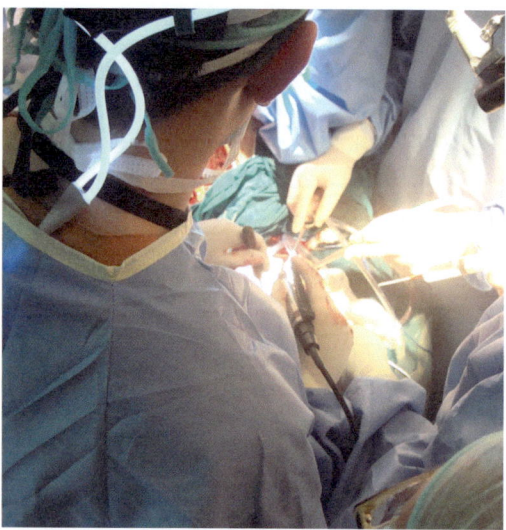

Fig. 13.4 Good organisation and leadership are necessary during simultaneous solid organs and face procurement. Note that there is not much room left during in situ dissection

The dissection proceeds until a final step is reached when the face graft is left attached either by the face skeleton and vessels or only by the vessel pedicles in case of a type A (no bone involved) face transplantation. During the whole dissection, all vessels, nerves and landmarks must be identified and marked for correct recipient's anastomosis and reconstruction. Haemostasis is also performed meticulously to minimise bleeding and instability during the whole procurement. It also prevents massive haemorrhage during revascularisation and recipient's reconstruction. At this moment, the dissection is stopped and all teams make them ready for preservation and final procurement of solid organs and grafts.

13.4.4 Final Step: Infusion and Procurement

Solid organ procurement with face VCA finalises with the infusion of preservation fluid and cooling. All teams are positioned either at the abdomen, thorax or cervicofacial area. Supporting staff make infusion pumps ready for perfusion of preservation and cardioplegic fluids. Lead transplant surgeon (multivisceral transplant surgeon in our institution) signals the start of cardioplegic infusion and preservation fluid infusion at 4 degrees Celsius. The donor is rapidly cooled down by direct application of sterile ice. We do not advise to apply sterile ice on face tissues but cooling them down with running infusion of Wisconsin (or similar) solution at 4 degrees Celsius. The operation finishes by section of major vessels, osteotomies if appropriate and indicated and section of any remaining attachments. If necessary, bank dissection (dissection with running solution on side sterile table in the operating room) is performed in the donor's theatre or adjacent operating room (in case of simultaneous bank dissection on different solid organs and face graft). The graft is then packed and dispatched in the standard manner to the recipient's operating room.

13.5   Face Graft Procurement: Surgical Technique

One should differentiate the surgical procurement of a face graft depending on the type of transplant planned. When only one part of the face is to be transplanted, the procurement dissection may be adapted to those anatomic landmarks. It is advised to procure some extra peripheral tissues in order to allow some room for adjustment at the time of graft insetting. However, in most face transplants (with plans for subtotal or total transplantation) a full-face graft shall be procured in order to make the final adjustment and trimming at the time of the recipient's insetting. During that part, a final decision whether some areas on the recipient's face should be ablated is then taken.

The operation begins with identification of major vessels in the neck (common carotid arteries and internal jugular veins). They are cannulated at this step if necessary. Care must be taken to plan the neck incision. It should match the incision in the recipient and allow for some extra skin for the postoperative skin biopsies. Cervical skin is undermined and dissected under the platysma muscle. The external carotid artery is identified and dissected. Major external carotid artery branches are identified and preserved if necessary for the type of face graft planned. In general terms, only the face artery is necessary for nearly all face transplants. Lingual artery is to be preserved if the tongue is included in the face transplant. Similarly, the hypoglossal nerve is identified, dissected and included in the transplant (face and tongue transplantation). The attention is then turned to the upper portion of the face graft to continue with the dissection.

13.5.1   Face Transplant Without Bone (Type A)

The operation follows in the upper portion of the graft. A bicoronal incision is performed. Dissection proceeds in the subperiosteal plane up to the level of the orbit. The supraorbital nerve is identified and dissected inside the orbit in order to lengthen it and allow for a tension-free neurorrhaphy. If a foramen is encountered, it is freed with chisel. Attention is directed to the lateral aspect of the face next. An incision is made at the appropriate level. If the ears are not included, a rhytidectomy incision is chosen. When the ears are transplanted, the incision is more posterior. The soft tissues are lifted and undermined. A deep dissection plane is employed, in order to include all face muscles and nerves. A more superficial plane is utilised when a type IV face transplant (skin and fat) is considered. All five face nerve branches are identified at the anterior margin of the parotid gland, cut and included in the graft. If the parotid gland is necessary for the face graft, it is included in the dissection. However, it increases the risk of postoperative sialocele. Care must be taken to include the Stensen's duct in continuity. The dissection approaches the infraorbital nerve and it is freed of adhesions. In order to achieve a long nerve stump, the floor of the orbit is opened and the nerve is identified in this position and severed. The nerve is then retracted with gentle traction. The masseter muscle marks the transition between the external layer and the full dissection of the cheek. If necessary, the mucosa and submucosa layers of the cheek are included with a full thickness dissection of the lips. Inferiorly, the dissection connects with the cervical flap. The dental nerve is identified at the mental foramen and severed and included in the flap. The final step during procurement consists of dissection and inclusion of the soft tissues and cartilages of the nose and section of the eyelids at the desired level. Current evidence supports vascularisation of full-face grafts through the face vessels that suffice for the entire face and face skeleton. Superficial temporal vessels may be included (at the preauricular level). Another option for the dissection of the vascular pedicle consists in the complete dissection of temporal vessels in continuity with the external carotid artery and the face artery. It does increase the level of complexity without evidence of improvement in vascularisation. The internal maxillary artery may be ligated in all types of transplants. Venous drainage includes the face, external jugular and anterior jugular vein or major tributaries. They may be dissected in continuity with the internal jugular if required.

13.5.2   Face Transplant Including Bone (Type B)

All general principles described in the previous section do apply for type B face graft procurement (see Figs. 13.5, 13.6, 13.7, 13.8, 13.9 and

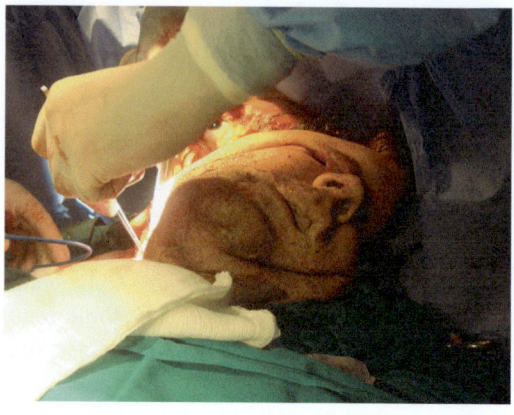

Fig. 13.7 Inferior dissection is directed to identify and prepare vessels and hypoglossal nerve if necessary. In type B flaps, the inferior border of the mandible is approached through a retromandibular route

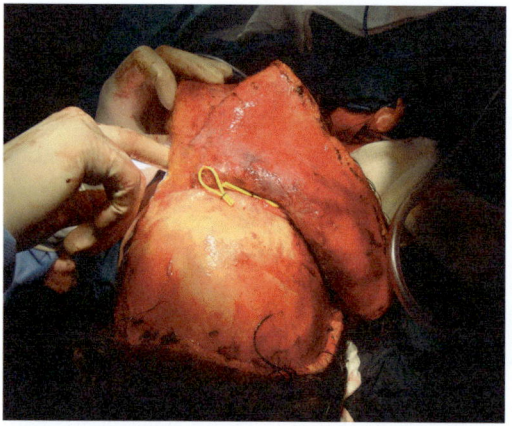

Fig. 13.5 Dissection of the superior part of the face proceeds in the subperiosteal plane to identify the supraorbital nerves

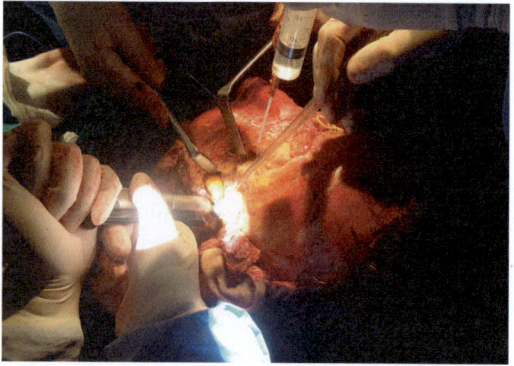

Fig. 13.8 Osteotomies are either performed before or after preservation fluid infusion. We recommend oscillating saws for good precision. Bone approaches depend on the type of transplant

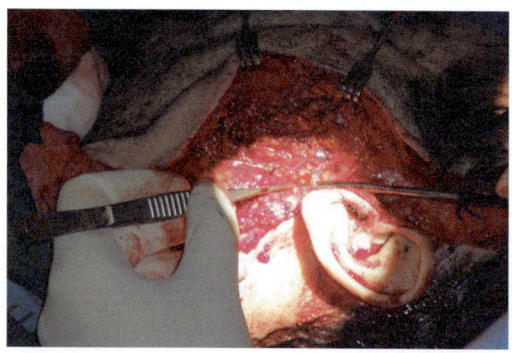

Fig. 13.6 Lateral dissection may include temporal vessels either in continuity or ligated at the parotid gland. Face nerve and main branches are identified and prepared for transplantation

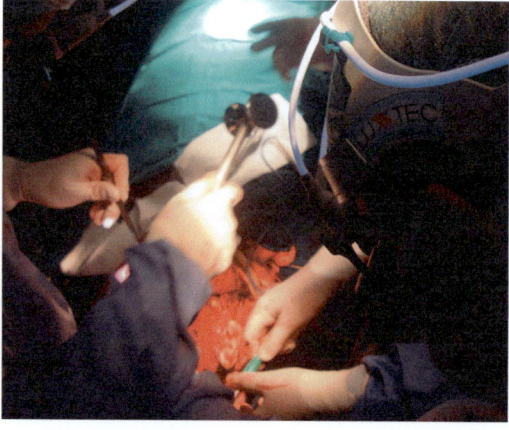

Fig. 13.9 Detachment of pterygoids and nasion (if necessary) with the aid of a chisel

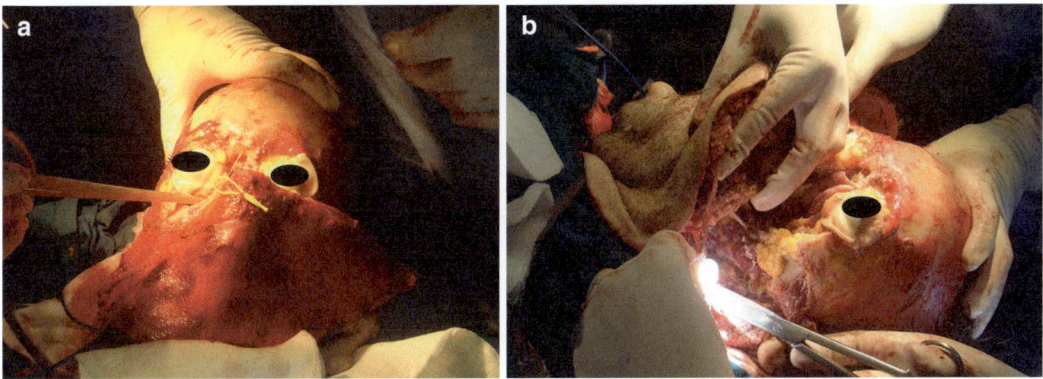

Fig. 13.10 (**a**, **b**) The final step of complete face degloving is posterior dissection (oropharynx or similar) dissection, perfusion and pedicle section

13.10). It follows the same vascular principles, although the retromandibular veins are also included in the flap. Good craniofacial expertise is necessary to perform a type B full-face transplant. Le Fort I, II or/and III osteotomies are normally planned, and so are mandibular osteotomies. They are selected and executed depending on the recipient's requirements. A well-defined operative plan is necessary with preoperative 3D angio-CT scans to prepare for a complex operation. Le Fort I, II or III osteotomies are performed with an oscillating saw and enter the orbit in a posterior curvilinear fashion. The infraorbital nerve is identified at this level and preserved. In order to complete the nasal osteotomy, the frontal flap is retracted inferiorly and the orbital periosteum elevated superiorly and medially. The nasion and the internal canthal ligaments mark the optimal level of osteotomy, which is connected with the orbital line of bony section. Next, the lateral flap is retracted medially, and osteotomy on the rest of the zygoma and the maxillary bone is performed. The pterygoids are detached with a chisel, and the whole mid-face is freed from the rest of the head.

After completion of the mid-face osteotomies and the soft tissue dissection, it allows for median distraction of the face en bloc, making room for medial mandibular dissection and identification of the dental nerve and lingual nerves at their origin in the skull base. They are dissected and cut in preparation for the recipient's neurorrhaphy.

The mandible is freed and dissected and the osteotomy is performed at the desired level. It is recommended to include extra length to perform the final adjustment in the recipient. Complete detachment of the mandible with the temporomandibular joint intact is also possible. The insertion of the median and lateral pterygoids and temporal muscles are severed and the final step includes dissection of the oropharynx at the desired level. At this step, the whole face, including the face skeleton, is fully detached and pedicled on the chosen blood vessels.

The procurement of face grafts can be tailored to the desired elements required for any given transplantation. Masseter muscles and nerves, parotid glands, tongue, oropharynx, ears, scalp, etc. may be included and the dissection protocol adapted. It is also recommended to create a specific plan and dissection schedule for each face transplant and to rehearse it in the anatomy dissection room. Similarly, each institution and transplant team should become proficient with different approaches and define their common technique for different face transplants. In our scenario, we do dissect and procure a full-face graft for all subtotal and total face transplants and only reserve partial approach when type III (eyelids) or type I (inferior) transplants are considered.

The inclusion of the tongue during face procurement calls for a specific approach during the inferior and mid-face dissection. As mentioned in the former section, median mandibular dissection shall identify a lingual nerve. During the cervical portion of the operation, lingual arteries and hypoglossal nerve are identified and freed to be included en bloc in the flap. The posterior margin of the dissection falls beyond the tongue base, including the epiglottis and the hypopharynx. We do advise to procure enough tissues that will allow for a tension-free and watertight suture.

13.6   Appendix 13.1: Informed Consent for the Donation of Face Allograft

Information that family and relatives of the donor must receive and understand:

1. You are being asked to donate the face structures of your relative (listed in section 3) for the transplantation of the face or parts of the face to reconstruct the face structures of a recipient (patient with severe face deformity). The recipient has been evaluated in a comprehensive manner by the face transplantation team and all reconstructive options have been taken into account. The transplantation of a full or partial face has remained the last and only option to reconstruct the face of the recipient. The face transplant team has proposed to utilise…*(list the parts of the face)*…of the face of another person (the donor).

2. The goals of this surgical intervention (the face transplantation) are:
   (a) Obtain a cosmetically acceptable face appearance.
   (b) Improve his/her quality of life.
   (c) Reassume a normal personal and social life interaction.

3. Apart from the internal organs (your transplant coordinator has informed you about solid organ donation separately), the following structures of the face will be obtained:
   (a) *List all that apply.*
   (b) *(…)*

4. The face appearance of the donor will not be maintained in the recipient after face transplantation. The aesthetics and face appearance depend on the face skeleton or part of it if bones are also transplanted. A new identity will be created, not resembling at all whatsoever the appearance of the donor.

5. Following donation and procurement of the donor's face or part of it, the face transplant team shall make every effort to restore the appearance of the donor by means of a custom-made face prosthesis, in order to preserve the dignity of the donor. You should anticipate, though, that the presentation of the cadaver will no longer be possible.

6. The face transplant team and all health workers involved in the donation and transplantation will preserve the intimacy of the donor's and recipient's family and shall make every effort to maintain their anonymous identity.

7. The medical team will publicly announce the face transplantation few days after the transplant has been completed in order to stimulate donations, to improve the knowledge of face deformity in society and to help future recipients and relatives for future transplantations.

8. The medical team involved in face transplantation does not receive any economic compensation by this type of reconstruction.
   Signed,
   Name and surname:
   Relationship with donor:
   Date:

Face Transplantation: Surgical Aspects

14

Abstract

Reconstructive allotransplantation has emerged as the ultimate restorative technique for treating face deformity, hand amputations and others. With the development of novel, more effective, immunosuppressant regimens, which shall decrease the advent of toxic side effects, the indication for this new technique may widen. In fact, the achievement of such a regimen that minimised side effects and counterbalanced the ethical issues in reconstructive allotransplantation would allow for the transplantation and restoration of any anatomical and functional unit of the human body. Cell therapy, tissue engineering and new synthetic polymers will help for the development of a true restorative surgery in the future, combining the knowledge and expertise of transplantation medicine with the advent and development of biological and synthetic tissue engineering.

14.1 Introduction

Reconstructive allotransplantation has emerged as the ultimate restorative technique for treating face deformity, hand amputations and others. With the development of novel, more effective, immunosuppressant regimens, which shall decrease the advent of toxic side effects, the indication for this new technique may widen. In fact, the achievement of such a regimen that minimised side effects and counterbalanced the ethical issues in reconstructive allotransplantation would allow for the transplantation and restoration of any anatomical and functional unit of the human body. Cell therapy, tissue engineering and new synthetic polymers will help for the development of a true restorative surgery in the future, combining the knowledge and expertise of transplantation medicine with the advent and development of biological and synthetic tissue engineering (Table 14.1).

The surgical treatment of face transplant patients follows the same principles and tenets observed in composite tissue transfer (free flaps) and craniofacial/maxillofacial surgery. A thorough study of the deformity and the health status of the patient is essential to make a global plan of treatment. All steps of the operation must be outlined, taking into consideration all difficult phases and creation of a strong multidisciplinary team. It is recommended that the recipient's operations be prepared and performed beforehand in the anatomy dissection room in order to avoid mistakes and unexpected errors during the operation.

J.P. Barret, V. Tomasello, *Face Transplantation: Principles, Techniques and Artistry*,
DOI 10.1007/978-3-662-45444-2_14, © Springer-Verlag Berlin Heidelberg 2015

The surgical team should prepare all details in order to be prepared for a continuous flow during the transplantation procedure. All surgical team members and anaesthesiologists must be well versed and have a complete knowledge of the whole procedure, since rotation of human resources during the transplantation phase is necessary to maintain safety during the surgical intervention. The main principles of face transplantation include the following:

- Organisation of the operating room and human resources
- Patient's preparation and induction therapy
- Extirpation of recipient's tissues

- Revascularisation
- Face transplantation
- Closure and patient's transfer

14.2   Organisation of the Operating Room and Human Resources

Large and spacious operating rooms are recommended for reconstructive allotransplantation. In general terms, rooms exceeding 40 square metres are advised. During face transplantation, a large number of transplantation teams are working together at the same time. It is not uncommon to join together at any given time two anaesthesiologist, two scrub nurses, four surgeons and two circulating nurses. Enough working space is necessary, to accommodate human resources and the necessary equipment (microscope, anaesthesia carts, instrumentarium, blood requirements, craniomaxillary instruments, etc.; see Fig. 14.1).

As soon as the team is warned that the transplant may be imminent, the head nurse should be informed in order to make ready all surgical instruments and blood products, prepare the OR

Table 14.1 Common principles of modern regenerative/restorative surgery

Cell therapy
Preservation and tissue modulation
Wound matrices and biomaterials
Immunological interaction
Engineered matrices and constructs
Transplantation medicine/immunomodulation principles

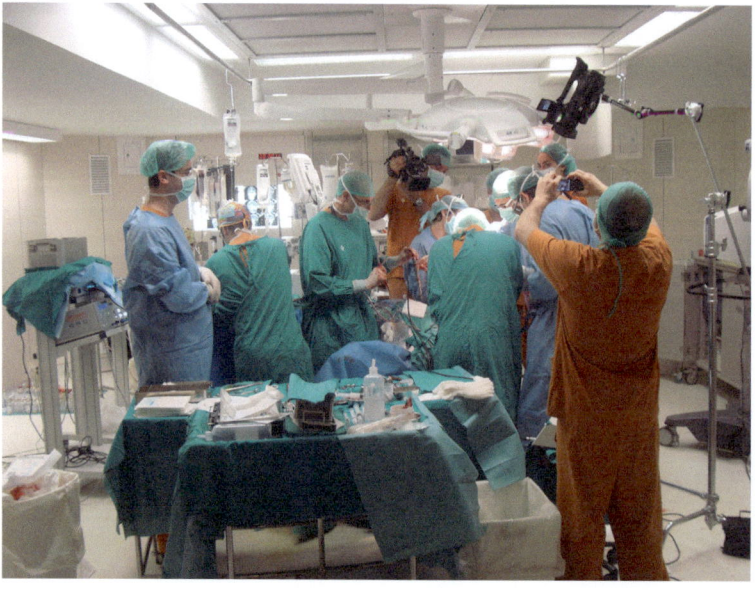

Fig. 14.1 Large and spacious theatre operating rooms are necessary for face transplantation. Microvascular instruments, microscopes, craniomaxillofacial instruments and others are common instruments during this type of procedures

nurse team and organise the shifts. It is advised to organise the team with two scrub nurses per shift and rotate them every 2–3 h. A total of 3–4 nurses may be necessary to provide enough rest during the procedure. In addition, the nursing team is completed with enough circulating personnel to provide external support.

Quick and thorough preparation of the anaesthesiology team is performed simultaneously. The head anaesthesiologist is informed of the proposed transplant procedure in order to make the team and the necessary material available. It is recommended that a minimum of two anaesthesiologists are present in the operating theatre at any given time. Major bleeding and difficult airway management is expected, and prompt decisions and manoeuvres may be necessary. In our experience, the anaesthesiology team should be completed with a third anaesthesiologist (minimum) in order to provide the necessary rest for the team. It is not uncommon for face transplantation procedures to last between 18 and 30 h. Under these circumstances, it is mandatory to rotate team members in order to maintain a safe environment and provide a good progress of the operation.

The surgical team should be formed by team players that are readily available all year round. Face transplantation is an urgent procedure that is carried out any time when a compatible multiple-organ donor is approached and informed consent from relatives is obtained. In comparison to other solid organ transplantation programmes, it is not feasible to have an on-call team on a 24-h basis, since donors are not commonly available and the number of patients in the waiting list for VCA is very low. Therefore, it is extremely important to build a strong team of enthusiastic surgeons that shall guarantee the successful development of a VCA procedure. Once the operation is planned, the team of surgeons should be organised in shifts, similarly to anaesthesia and nursing teams. Our approach consists of three to four plastic surgeons per shift (depending on the complexity of the phase of the operation) that rotate every 2–3 h (Table 14.2). The team leader takes the responsibility to organise all rotations and it is his/her responsibility to oversee the good progression of the operation. It is advisable to name an assistant team leader in order to provide the necessary rest for the team leader at any given time. The master plan for the operation should be outlined before the patient is taken to operation room and all difficult points revised.

Table 14.2 Recommended rotation of team members

Anaesthesia:
2 anaesthesiologists on site; rotate every 3–4 h
Minimum of 3 anaesthesiologists
Surgeons:
3–4 surgeons on site; rotate every 2–3 h
Minimum of 6–8 surgeons
Scrub nurses:
2 scrub nurses; rotate every 2–3 h
Minimum of 3–4 nurses

The head anaesthesiologist, head nurse and team leader must revise and make sure that all necessary equipment, materials, blood products and necessary support from other services are ready and available before the recipient is taken to the operating room. Other necessary and mandatory team members include transplant coordinators (at least one coordinator should be present during the whole procedure), infectious diseases/immunologists and transplant surgeons (these team members shall help in infectious disease prophylaxis, induction immunosuppressant therapy and technical pitfalls during the transplantation). It is not absolutely necessary that they are present in the operating room, although it is mandatory that they can be reached within minutes. Other support services include porters, housekeeping, ward nurses, pharmacy, mass media coordination and tissue/blood banking. The rest of the team members (Table 14.3) should be informed of an imminent transplant since their assistance will be necessary from day 1.

The organisation of the operating room within the hospital differs depending on the type of the expected donation. If the donor is located in the same hospital, our advice is to follow the Boston approach if possible: the donor's and recipient's operating rooms should be run in parallel. With this approach, the graft is procured in the operating room next door, and it can be transported within seconds to the recipient's room (which is normally located a few metres on the room next door). With this organisation, complex and cumbersome packaging in a container with preservation fluid is avoided and the graft is manipulated as any other routine free flap. Once the VCA graft is detached from the donor (after preservation fluid infusion), the graft is transported to the recipient's site in the standard fashion. If this approach is selected, one must remember, though, that a third parallel room (on the other side of the donor's theatre) may be required to perform bank surgery on solid organs (Fig. 14.2). This approach, when feasible, saves time and helps with the organisation and coordination of both the donor's and the recipient's transplant teams. On the other hand, if the donor

is not located in the same hospital or, given the architecture of the hospital (commonly in health science centres, when different hospitals form the complex), the donation must be contemplated as a distant donor, both the donor's and recipient's theatres being distant and the transportation of the VCA graft must be performed in a container with preservation fluid and secured and transferred to the recipient's operation room as in any standard solid organ transplantation procedure. When this approach has to be implemented, cold ischaemia time should be kept to a minimum and the organisation and coordination of both teams is much more complicated. Direct communication between both theatres' teams is essential to couple both surgeries; as soon as the procurement process is considered to progress in good condition, the recipient's team should start the procedure to induce the immunosuppressant protocol, secure the airway and prepare the recipient's vessels.

Table 14.3 Organisation of face VCA team

1. Chief surgeon (team leader)
2. Plastic surgeons
3. Transplant surgeons
4. Transplant coordinators
5. Immunologist
6. Infectious disease specialist
7. Psychiatrist
8. Psychologist
9. Pathologist
10. Nephrologists
11. Surgical critical-care specialist
12. Nurses
13. Mass media relations coordinators
14. Rehabilitation services
15. Speech pathologist
16. Dietician
17. Pharmacists
18. Support services

14.3 Patient Preparation and Induction Therapy

Following the activation of the face VCA team and the thorough evaluation of the donor, with confirmation of the compatibility of the patient's characteristics and full informed consent, the donor is confirmed and the recipient is contacted. As soon as the patient arrives to the hospital, a complete preoperative check is carried out (Table 14.4), including cross-match and blood typing to order the necessary blood products. Preoperative pictures are obtained and the

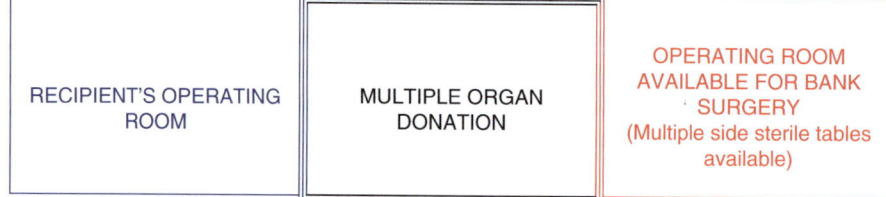

Fig. 14.2 Common organisation of parallel operating rooms for VCA procedures. Simultaneous operating rooms may be added in case transplantation of solid organs is planned in the same institution

Table 14.4 Preoperative checklist

1. Complete blood test and coagulation panel
2. Contact infectious disease specialist
3. CMV and EPV serologies (if negative)
4. Type and screen blood analysis and order blood products
5. PRA (not necessary if less than 3 months from previous test)
6. Tissue typing
7. Prophylactic antibiotics (check with infectious diseases)
8. Chest X-ray
9. Blood, urine, pharynx, tracheostomy microbiological cultures
10. Contact anaesthesiology department
11. If PRA > 50 %, IV IgG 2 g/kg
12. Thymoglobulin 2 mg/kg; premedicate 30 min before infusion with 1 g prednisone, Benadryl 50 mg/IV, acetaminophen 650 mg

Table 14.5 Induction immunosuppression regime

1. Thymoglobulin 2 mg/kg[a]
2. Premedicate 30 min before with
(a) Infusion with 1 g prednisone
(b) Benadryl 50 mg/IV
(c) Acetaminophen 650 mg

[a]Other anti-lymphocyte or anti-cytokine antibodies may be used

procedure is reviewed and outlined with the patient. In our practice informed consent is obtained during the general evaluation of patients. It is one of the most important items in ethical committee evaluation. Consequently, it cannot be changed or modified at this stage without the committee not being informed. Readers are referred to their local regulatory body for counselling. Surgeons are advised to update informed consents if their regulatory body do accept this practice. The patient is admitted and accommodated in his/her room until the donor's team informs the recipient's team whether the operation may proceed or not. In case the allograft cannot be successfully transplanted, the patient is discharged home and he/she returns to the exact position in the waiting list. On the other hand if the allograft can be transplanted, the patient is then taken to the recipient's operating theatre.

As soon as the patient arrives to the operating room, the patient is positioned in the operating table, and all comfort measures are implemented. A long operation is expected; thus, all preventive actions to prevent pressure sores and deep venous thrombosis should be followed. Central lines, large bore IV lines and arterial lines are advised. We recommend placing them after the induction of the anaesthesia. It is our practice to administer the induction immunosuppressant drugs in the operating room after the induction of the anaesthesia (Table 14.5). In this fashion, the patient is well controlled and placed in a safe environment should any adverse event of the medications occur.

The final step of this phase consists in securing the patient's airway. We advise to secure the airway by means of a surgical tracheotomy. It can be safely perform after the induction of the anaesthesia. On the other hand, if the patient has a tracheotomy in place, the cannula is replaced by a wider diameter and affixed with stitches. Similarly, if percutaneous gastric tube feeding is contemplated (and the patient has no PEG tube in place), it is introduced by the endoscopy department during this phase of the operation.

14.4   Extirpation of the Recipient's Tissues

The patient is prepped and dressed in the standard sterile fashion, following head and neck principles. We recommend preparing both thighs in case great saphenous vein grafts are necessary.

An incision is made at the midpoint of the neck as a standard bilateral neck dissection. The main arteries and veins in the neck are dissected, exposed and prepared. All main branches of the external carotid artery should also be identified and prepared for a possible anastomosis. We recommend an end-to-end anastomosis of the external carotid artery in full-face allografts, although they may also survive with a bilateral face artery anastomosis and temporal anastomosis if necessary. Depending on the recipient's anastomosis and deformity, vein grafts and/or loops may be required (in those cases when some vessels have been destroyed by the accident/deformity or have been used in previous reconstructions).

At this stage two approaches are possible:
1. Revascularisation, followed by recipient's face extirpation or
2. Recipient's face extirpation and revascularisation

One should remember that the resection of the recipient's face is a point of no return. Following the extirpation of the face, the only restorative option is a face transplantation. Hence, our advice in all face transplantations is to perform allograft revascularisation followed by the recipient's face extirpation. However, both alternatives are possible and render excellent outcomes. One must remember, though, that if one opts to revascularise and extirpate the recipient's face afterwards, vein grafts may be necessary and the operation may turn much more complex.

The extirpation of the recipient's face structures follows the same phases similar to the procurement of face allografts. The same areas that have been obtained in the donor are resected, paying attention to detail and preserving nerves and vessels that will be necessary for a successful transplantation. General principles of head and neck surgery and craniomaxillary surgery are necessary for a correct resection (Fig. 14.3). The operation may start from an inferior or superior approach. As soon as the central portion of the face is reached, the opera-

tion is then turned to both lateral areas, until the whole specimen is detached from the deep structures and the face skeleton (Fig. 14.4). Sensory and motor nerves are identified and prepared for neurorrhaphy. The rest of the structures that are necessary for correct restoration of anatomy are tailored at this stage. All necessary osteotomies are performed, leaving the defect ready for transplantation. When this step of the operation is reached, the whole deformed anatomy of the recipient has been resected and the resulting defect mimics the donor's final operation result. The rest of the area is prepared for the reconstruction and all nerves, vessels and other relevant structures identified and tagged (Fig. 14.5).

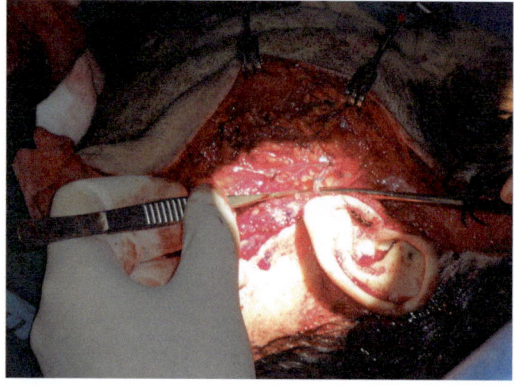

Fig. 14.3 Extirpation of recipient's face tissues follows a similar approach of the donor's allograft procurement

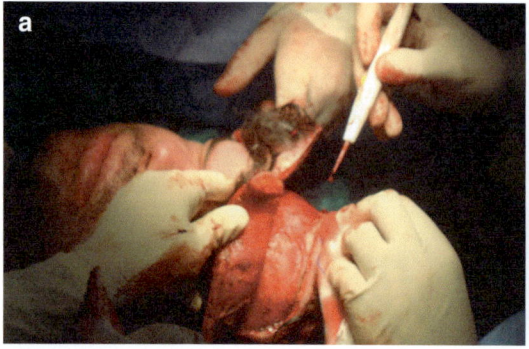
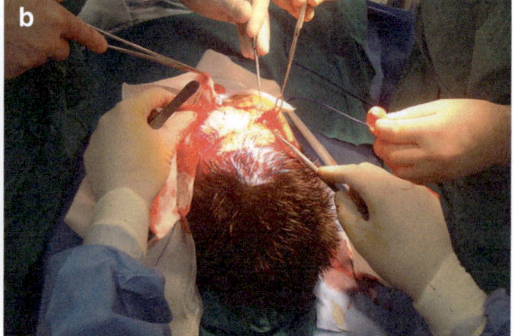

Fig. 14.4 After careful homeostasis (**a**), the defect is trimmed (**b**) to match that in the donor operation to provide a perfect reconstruction

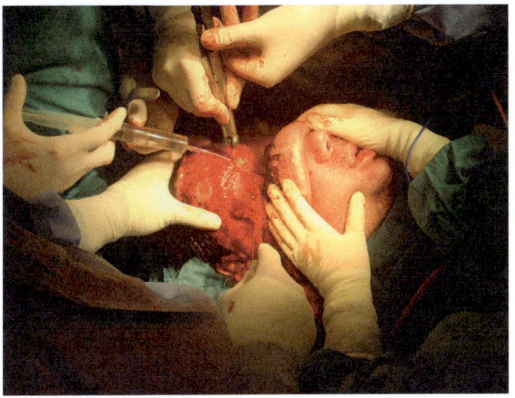

Fig. 14.5 Osteotomies during full-face allotransplantation

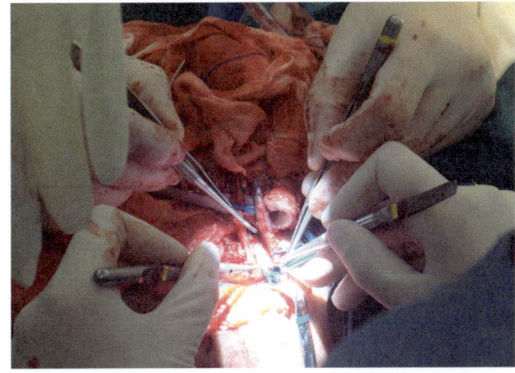

Fig. 14.6 Direct revascularisation with vein grafts of face allograft in the neck

14.5 Revascularisation

Timing of revascularisation depends on the approach to face transplantation adopted by the transplantation team. Revascularisation before face extirpation is more complex (Fig. 14.6). The recipient's operation must proceed with the face allograft in vicinity which forces for multiple manoeuvres. In this situation haemostasis is more difficult and vein grafts are normally necessary. When revascularisation is performed after face extirpation, allograft adaptation is less complex and vein grafts are not necessary in many instances since the allograft is inset after revascularisation. However, ischaemia time is prolonged which may pose some problems in terms of ischaemia–reperfusion injury. General advice calls for a rapid revascularisation to shorten as much as possible ischaemia time. However, other VCA experiences (limb transplantation) have also proved that prolonged ischaemia time (at the end of the transplantation after all bones, nerves and tendons have been reconstructed) does not increase infection, tissue necrosis or ischaemia–reperfusion injury. The team should evaluate the difficulty of the tissue resection and adapt the time of revascularisation to it. An alternative to limit ischaemia time that allows a less complex face resection is revascularisation at a distant site in the recipient as a bridge to final anastomosis in the face. This temporal anastomosis may be performed in the

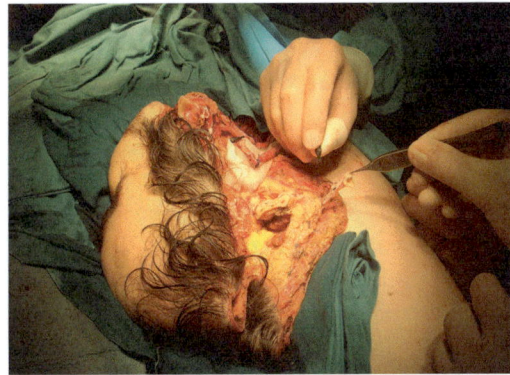

Fig. 14.7 Revascularisation of a face allograft in the groin. The use of vein grafts facilitates this technique

inguinal area, between the femoral vessels and the face recipient vessels by using vein grafts (Fig. 14.7). Ischaemia time is shortened by this temporal revascularisation, although it increases the risk of ischaemia–reperfusion injury by performing the anastomosis twice after a period of intact circulation.

Regardless of the time and type of revascularisation, it is necessary to infuse 1 g of prednisone IV just before clamps are released and the tissues perfused anew. It decreases the release of cytokines, inflammation and any immune reactions from HLA mismatches and other antigens and the preservation fluid metabolic disturbances. After revascularisation, new tissue biopsies are obtained from skin and mucosa in order to have background biopsies (Fig. 14.8).

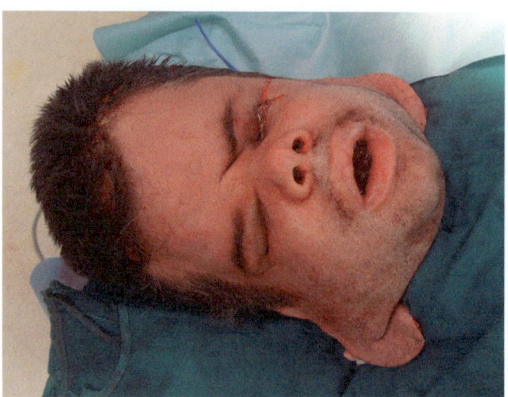

Fig. 14.8 Following revascularisation, a complete hyperaemic appearance is expected. At this moment background skin and mucosa biopsies are obtained

Table 14.6 General organisation of face transplantation surgery involving bones (if applicable)

1. Trimming and preparation of recipient face
2. Temporary inset of the allograft
3. Suture of intraoral structures
4. Mandibular nerve neurorrhaphy
5. Infraorbital nerve neurorrhaphy
6. Miniplate osteosynthesis and intermaxillary fixation
7. Supraorbital nerve neurorrhaphy
8. Face nerve neurorrhaphy
9. Hypoglossal nerve neurorrhaphy
10. Soft tissue suture and skin

14.6   Face Transplantation

The transplantation of face allografts should be attempted in a step-by-step manner. As mentioned before, principles of head and neck reconstruction and craniomaxillofacial surgery do apply. Depending on the type of face transplant, the course of the operation may vary, although a general organisation of the operation (Table 14.6) is indicated to all of them.

Face allografts and recipients are sufficiently trimmed and prepared for correct adaptation of all tissues. Few temporal insets are performed during this stage to prepare the allograft. At this moment bones are also adapted and osteotomies performed if indicated to allow for a correct bony alignment at the time of bone synthesis (Fig. 14.9). As soon as the allograft and the recipient face tissues are fully prepared, the final inset begins.

Face allograft inset starts with a water seal suture of all intraoral structures, similarly to that executed in head and neck reconstruction. If the tongue is included in the transplant, it is also inset and fixated to the remainder of the recipient's sutures. All muscles are sutured together to allow for a correct functional outcome. Following this initial step, attention is turned to the mandibular, lingual and hypoglossal nerves, which lie deep in the parapharyngeal area. These nerves must be

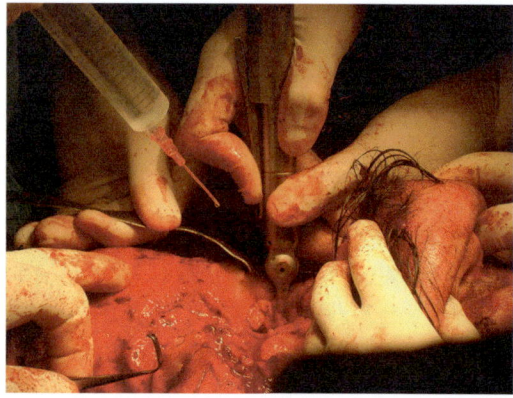

Fig. 14.9 Trimming soft tissues and bone elements is necessary for correct alignment of the face allograft

anastomosed before the face skeleton is affixed, in order to get good access. If the bony skeleton is aligned and fixated with miniplates, nerves may lie in a deep and non-accessible position. A similar action is necessary for the infraorbital nerve. When the face bones are transplanted, the nerve anastomosis is performed below the floor of the orbit. This structure is only accessible before osteosynthesis is performed, when the whole allograft is mobile and may be reached on both sides.

Face bone osteosynthesis are performed in the standard fashion (Fig. 14.10a, b). The same techniques and principles of maxillofacial surgery are indicated and employed. The usual osteotomy lines will follow standard Le Fort I, Le Fort II and Le Fort III fractures. In the mandibular area, the osteotomy

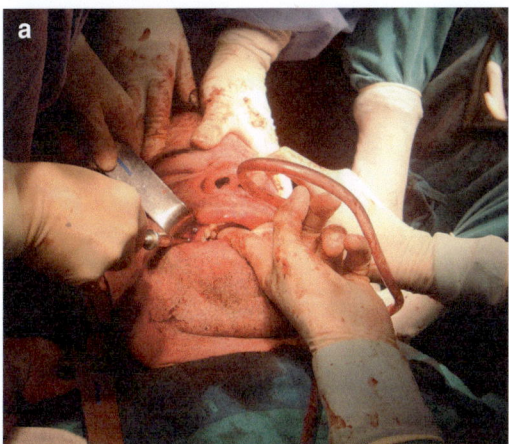

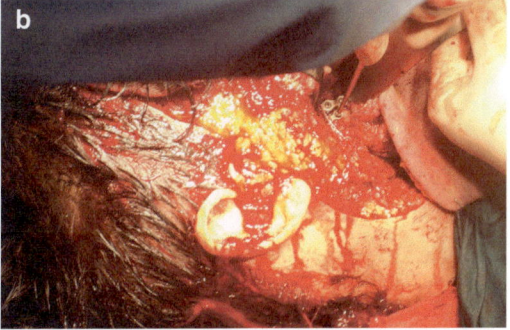

Fig. 14.10 (**a, b**) Miniplate osteosynthesis are performed in the same manner utilised in craniomaxillofacial operations

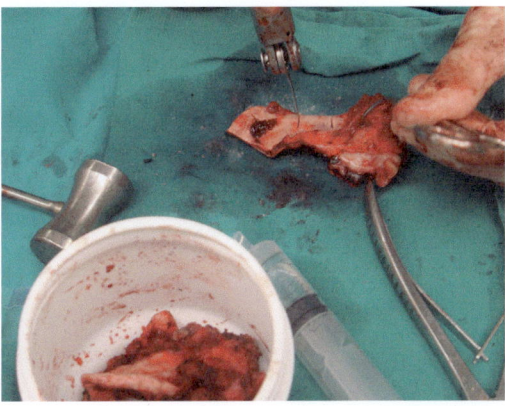

Fig. 14.11 Recipient's bones resected during face transplant preparation may serve as a source of bone grafts during allograft inset

lines lie following standard orthognathic surgery bone cuts. Rigid titanium miniplates are utilised for osteosynthesis, which are presented in different widths and lengths and may be tailored for each individual case. We advise to harvest and keep in saline all resected bones from the recipient for their utilisation as bone grafts, avoiding an extra donor site in the recipient (Fig. 14.11). We do not advise to use any biomaterial at this stage since this type of materials may not be well integrated and promote infection in an otherwise immunocompromised patient. This part of the operation is completed with intermaxillary fixation with occlusion screws and elastic bands if necessary. We recommend to avoid fixation unless absolutely necessary; oral hygiene may be compromised and feeding complications difficult to treat and prevent.

Eyelids, canthal ligaments and tendons, orbicularis muscles, levator aponeurosis and con-

junctiva are restored next. These structures must be sutured and restored before the supraorbital nerve is anastomosed. If the nose, including the nasal bones, is transplanted, the medial canthal ligament and the lachrymal apparatus are intact in the allograft, and there is no need to perform any extra manoeuvre for their reconstruction. However, if the bony skeleton is not transplanted in the nasal area, the lachrymal apparatus must be cannulated and restored, together with the medial canthal ligament and tendon. The supraorbital nerve neurorrhaphy is performed after all periorbital structures have been restored and reconstructed. The rest of the deep structures in the mid-face are sutured and restored (i.e. masseter muscle, Stensen's duct, etc.). As mentioned before, every essential ligament, anatomic landmark, etc., in this area medial to the face branches have to be sutured and reconstructed before the final face nerve stage of the operation is reached. Following these neurorrhaphies, they will be no longer accessible.

Attention is then turned to the face nerve. All nerves (identified and tagged previously, see Fig. 14.12) are anastomosed in the standard fashion. Nerve grafts are normally not necessary (Fig. 14.13). The muscles are then approximated and the rest of the face ligaments restored to help with sphincter and soft tissue retention.

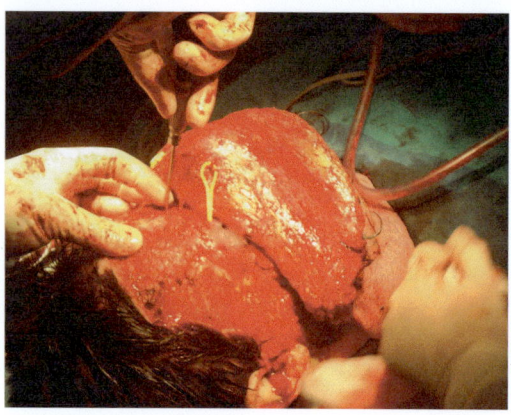

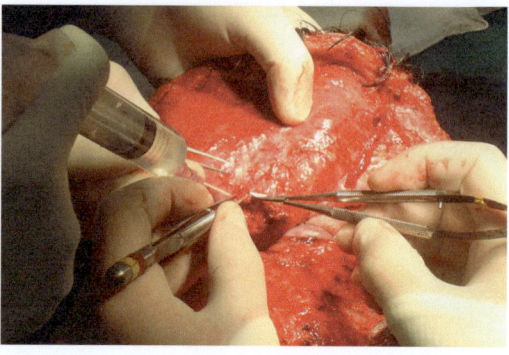

Fig. 14.13 Face nerve branches neurorrhaphies are one of the few last steps of face transplantation. Many of the structures of the face allograft will not be accessible after this neurorrhaphies

Fig. 14.12 All nerves and other structures are tagged in preparation for correct and rapid anastomosis

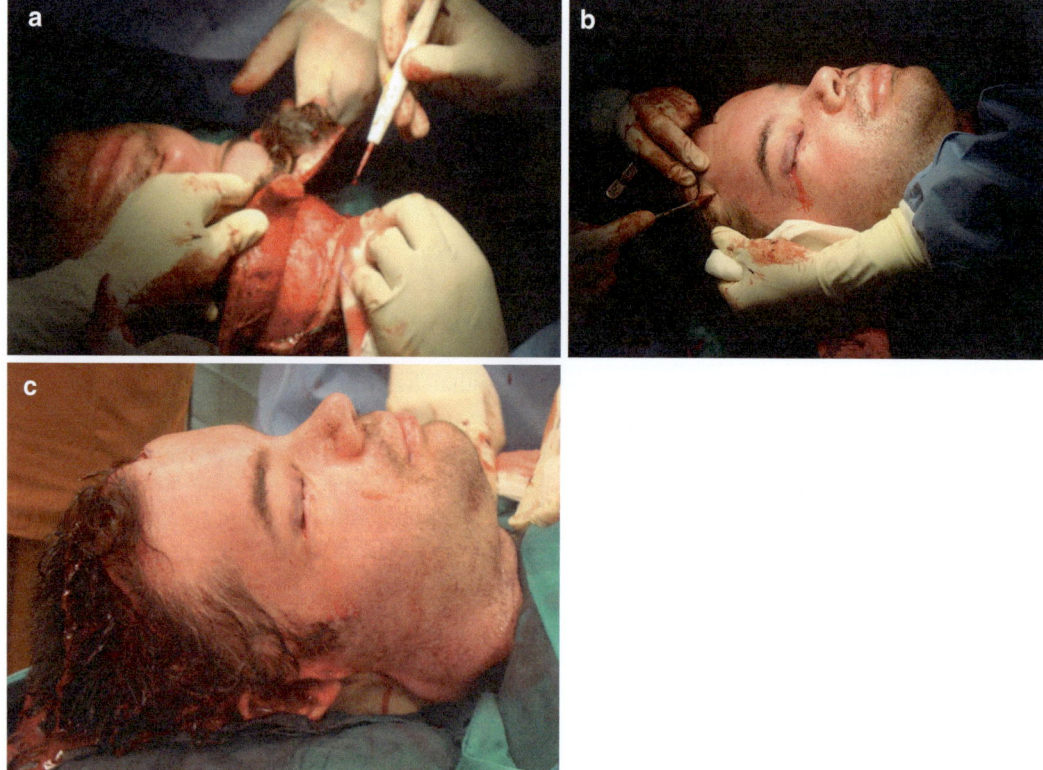

Fig. 14.14 (**a–c**) Face skin and soft tissues excess are trimmed in order to obtain good allograft adaptation

14.7 Closure and Patient's Transfer

The final stages of face transplantation follow similar techniques and steps as any other face reconstructive operation. Soft tissues are approx-

imated and any excess trimmed (Fig. 14.14a–c). It is recommended to allow for some excess in the most lateral or inferior aspect of the allograft for tissue biopsies. In this manner, scars and marks are concealed to hidden areas that may be extirpated at the end of the first year posttransplant. Suction drains are introduced as needed depending on the type of transplanted areas. Surgeons may decide to use any fibrin sealant available, which shall prevent seroma and other complications. All sutures and transplanted areas are left exposed for good postoperative control. The patient is then ready for transfer to the intensive care unit. The standard immunosuppressant protocol is started, and the patient is controlled following ICU protocols. We recommend weaning off the ventilator during the following hours and having a complete alert and awake patient within 24 h after surgery. Feeding is started via the enteral route immediately. Oral intake is started as soon as the patient clinical situation dictates to do so. The patient is inspected hourly for vascularisation, colour, temperature and Doppler signal. Superficial temperature probes are also useful. The local allograft flap control does not differ much from the usual microvascular flap monitoring. We recommend taking daily photographs for postoperative control of rejection. The patient is allowed to see his/her new appearance as soon as he/she requests to do so with the support of the psychology–psychiatric team.

14.8   Appendix 14.1: Postoperative Orders

1. Diagnosis.
2. Check vital signs according to ICU protocol.
3. Check fluid balance every hour.
4. Tracheotomy care as per ICU protocol.
5. Central line management as per ICU protocol.
6. Nihl by mouth (exception, oral medications).
7. NG tube to gravity.
8. Urinary catheter and control of hourly urine output.
9. Check drains every 2 h.
10. Chest X-ray on admission to ICU.
11. Control of anastomosis with hand-held Doppler every hour for the first 24 h and then every 2 h for 6 days.
12. Blood test on admission to ICU:

(a) Blood gas analysis with lactate and calcium (ion)
(b) Complete blood cell count, platelets, prothrombin and partial thromboplastin ratios, fibrinogen, AST, ALT, bilirubin, GGTP, calcium/magnesium/phosphate, sodium/potassium/chlorine, total proteins, BUN, creatinine and glucose
13. Daily blood test:
(a) Complete blood cell count, platelets, prothrombin and partial thromboplastin ratios, fibrinogen, AST, ALT, bilirubin, GGTP, calcium/magnesium/phosphate, sodium/potassium/chlorine, total proteins, albumin, BUN, creatinine, glucose and tacrolimus level
14. Cross-match on first day posttransplant.
15. IV fluids as per protocol ICU and patient response.
16. IV broad-spectrum antibiotics according to institution guidelines (cover Gram + cocci and Gram– bacteria):
(a) Continue 3–5 days.
(b) Change to appropriate antibiotics when surveillance microbiological results from donor and recipients are available (or PCRs).
17. Antifungal prophylaxis (liposome amphotericin, 1 mg/kg IV).
18. Trimethoprim/sulfamethoxazole IV every 24 h until good oral tolerance; start then 80 mg PO three times per week.
19. Ganciclovir 5 mg/kg bid until good oral tolerance (if recipient– and donor+).
20. Tacrolimus 0.15 mg/kg/24 h IV in perfusion 24 h; switch to PO when good oral intake and correct iv levels.
21. Thymoglobulin 2 mg/kg IV in IV perfusion (over 12 h). Premedicate patients 30 min before administration with prednisone 2 mg/kg, Benadryl 1 mg/kg and acetaminophen 10 mg/kg.
22. Prednisone 2 mg/kg/day.
23. Topical tacrolimus 0.1 % 2 times per day for 2 months (start 10 days postoperative).
24. Mycostatin oral rinses every 8 h.
25. Omeprazole 40 mg/24 h.
26. AAS 100 mg PO every 24 h (3 weeks).

27. Low molecular heparin s.c. when platelet count >100,000.
28. Check capillary glucose every 6 h.
29. Insulin in sliding scale.
30. In case of rejection, start protocol (boluses of methylprednisolone) followed by daily quick taper:
    (a) First day, 5 mg/kg/day = _____ mg IV Q 6 h (divided in 4 doses)
    (b) Second day, 4 mg/kg/day = _____ mg IV Q 6 h (divided in 4 doses)
    (c) Third day, 3 mg/kg/day = _____ mg IV Q 6 h (divided in 4 doses)
    (d) Fourth day, 2 mg/kg/day = _____ mg IV Q 6 h (divided in 4 doses)
    (e) Fifth day, 2 mg/kg/day = _____ mg IV Q 12 h (divided in 2 doses); continued overtime mandated by clinical course

A General Overview of Current Outcomes

Abstract

Face transplantation is a new achievement of transplantation medicine and microvascular reconstructive plastic surgery. However, the initial ethical and technical debate was not less intense, which tried to balance advantages and disadvantages of face transplantation. It was clear from the initial discussion at the beginning of the year 2000 that certain cases could benefit for such an approach, although real functional outcomes lacked support from ethical committees. More than ever, a continuous surveillance and detailed outcomes are necessary to put into perspective the indications and contraindications of face transplantation.

The modern history of vascularised composite tissue allotransplantation began in 1998, when the first human hand transplantation became a reality. Few years afterwards, in 2005, the first human face transplantation was attempted with success by Devauchelle and Dubernard in France.

Face transplantation is a new achievement of transplantation medicine and microvascular reconstructive plastic surgery. However, the initial ethical and technical debate was not less intense, which tried to balance advantages and disadvantages of face transplantation. It was clear from the initial discussion at the beginning of the year 2000 that certain cases could benefit for such an approach, although real functional outcomes lacked support from ethical committees. More than ever a continuous surveillance and detailed outcomes are necessary to put into perspective the indications and contraindications of face transplantation.

To date, 28 face transplantations have been performed worldwide. Medicine is an ever-evolving science, and as such, at the time this work comes to the public, it is certain that new and novel face transplantations shall be attempted. The reader is therefore advised to keep updated with VCA literature and from reports from the international society of hand and composite tissue allotransplantation. Face VCA refers to allografts that contain different tissues (bone, muscle, skin, fat, mucosa, vessels); they are vascularised by one or many vascular pedicles, and in order to survive, the same principles that apply to solid organ transplantation should be followed.

15.1   Worldwide Experience on Face Transplantation

Twenty-eight face transplants have been performed in seven countries (Table 15.1). The longest follow-up period accounts for 8 years (Isabelle Dinoire, Amiens team) with a total published survival rate of 89.3 %. Three patients have died (1 patient in China, 1 patient in France-Paris team, 1 patient in Spain-Valencia team). Table 15.2 depicts transplant characteristics. Fourteen different transplant teams have performed in total 17 partial-face transplants and 11 full-face transplants for a variety of aetiologies that include 10 postburn deformities, 8 gunshot injuries, 3 animal attacks, 4 type 1 neurofibromatosis, 2 posttraumatic deformities and 1 postoncological/radiotherapy deformities. After the transplantation of the first full-face transplant in 2010, the indications have expanded; however, a robust team approach and specific face VCA protocols are necessary to warrant correct outcomes. The indications for face transplantation vary among different VCA teams. In general terms, destruction of face sphincters (orbital and/or oral muscle sphincters) is a common indication for face transplantation (there currently does not exist a traditional technique that repair the function of such sphincters). Contraindications include significant medical co-morbidities, poor adhesion to medical follow-up, medical risk for immunosuppressant therapy (recurrent cancer,

medical co-morbidities regarding past medical history) and psychological/psychiatric instability. Most of the patients have undergone previous reconstruction by traditional techniques, although there is intense debate whether face transplantation should be performed early in the hospital course to leave intact other traditional techniques and donor sites should the transplanted graft failed. Most of the teams performed procurement on a brain-dead heart-beating donor. Some teams advocate to procure the face before the rest of the solid organs are approached, although synchronous procurement is feasible, as it has been reported by our team. It is imperative to reduce cold ischaemia time during VCA. Some teams procured the face VCA at the end of the procedure (i.e. Chinese, Valencia's, and Seville's teams); this approach, though, may lead to a massive haemorrhage after revascularisation and increase the risk of ischaemia–reperfusion injury.

15.2   Type of Transplants

The composition of the different face VCA graft varies and depends on the recipient's requirements (Table 15.2). In half of the cases, the bone has been transplanted as part of the face transplant graft, most of which included the maxilla and mandible (especially in gunshot injuries and trauma cases). Open rigid miniplate fixation, similarly to that utilised in craniomaxillary surgery, has been employed with excellent results. Survival of all tissues included in the transplanted specimen has been observed. There is no contraindication regarding the type of transplanted tissues. The experience gathered from all face transplants performed to date warrants good perfusion and postoperative results regardless of the type of transplant to be performed. All teams advise, though, to make some experimental dissection in the anatomy lab to improve the efficiency of the transplant process. It is imperative to perform a good

Table 15.1 Worldwide experience of face transplantation

Country	Number of centres	Total number of face VCAs per country
France	2	9
USA	3	7
Turkey	2	5
Spain	3	3
Poland	1	2
Belgium	1	1
China	1	1

Table 15.2 World's experience on face VCA to date

Number	Date	Team	Type	Aetiology	Outcome
1	11/2005	Amiens, France	Partial	Animal attack	Alive
2	04/2006	Xian, China	Partial+bone	Animal attack	Patient died
3	01/2007	Paris, France	Partial	Neurofibromatosis	Alive
4	12/2008	Cleveland, USA	Partial+bone	Gunshot injury	Alive
5	03/2009	Paris, France	Partial+bone	Gunshot injury	Alive
6	04/2009	Paris, France	Partial	Burn	Patient died
7	08/2009	Boston, USA	Partial+bone	Burn	Alive
8	08/2009	Paris, France	Partial+bone	Gunshot injury	Alive
9	08/2009	Valencia, Spain	Partial+bone	Postoncological+ radiotherapy	Patient died
10	11/2009	Amiens, France	Partial+bone	Burn	Alive
11	01/2010	Seville, Spain	Partial	Neurofibromatosis	Alive
12	03/2010	Barcelona, Spain	Full+bone	Gunshot injury	Alive
13	07/2010	Paris, France	Full	Neurofibromatosis	Alive
14	03/2011	Boston, USA	Full	Burn	Alive
15	04/2011	Paris, France	Partial+bone	Gunshot injury	Alive
16	04/2011	Paris, France	Partial+bone	Gunshot injury	Alive
17	04/2011	Boston, USA	Full	Burn	Alive
18	05/2011	Boston, USA	Full	Animal attack	Alive
19	01/2012	Antalya, Turkey	Full+bone	Burn	Alive
20	01/2012	Gent, Belgium	Partial+bone	Trauma	Alive
21	02/2012	Ankara, Turkey	Full	Burn	Alive
22	03/2012	Ankara, Turkey	Partial	Burn	Alive
23	03/2012	Baltimore, USA	Full+bone	Gunshot injury	Alive
24	05/2012	Antalya, Turkey	Full	Burn	Alive
25	01/2013	Boston, USA	Full	Burn	Alive
26	05/2013	Antalya, Turkey	Partial+bone	Gunshot injury	Alive
27	07/2013	Gliwice, Poland	Partial+bone	Trauma	Alive
28	12/2013	Gliwice, Poland	Full	Neurofibromatosis	Alive

preoperative inspection of intraoral structures since any chronic infection (especially in the dental area) may pose a significant risk for the recipient.

15.3 Revascularisation

Good perfusion and face viability has been observed in all cases. The whole face can be successfully revascularised by one face artery (including the maxilla and mandible through network connections and periosteal feeders), although all teams advocate for a bilateral arterial anastomosis to ensure safety. In general terms, large arterial vessels are employed (external carotid artery). Some teams have performed extensive anatomic clinical research which shows that correct vascularisation do occur through the face artery system. A consensus does exist that temporal vessels may not be necessary in most of the face transplants and should be considered only in cases with large portions of the scalp and external auricle. The preferred method to study the recipient's vascular status includes angio-CT scan, which provides not only information of the arterial and venous network but also a good exploration of the face skeleton and the bone–soft tissue relationship.

15.4   Nerve Recovery

The main objective of face transplantation is improvement of function and quality of life and reintegration into society as full individuals. Therefore, sensation and motor function play a central role to achieve the main goal of face VCA. Motor nerve reinnervation is necessary to achieve correct function when face transplantation is indicated for improvement in function and face muscles, masticator muscles or tongue is transplanted. End-to-end neurorrhaphies are performed by all transplant teams between face nerve branches, motor branches of the trigeminal nerve and hypoglossal nerve. As soon as 3 months after surgery patients may experience fasciculations and a progressive improvement in muscle tone, although it is not until 6–12 months after transplantation that active movements are apparent. Complete recovery of all face muscle movement seldom does occur, and a progressive recovery of function is observed that prolongs more than 24 months posttransplant. Sensation appears earlier in the postoperative course. As soon as 2–3 months posttransplant, patients may feel in their new faces, and complete sensory recovery is apparent 12 months after transplant. Surprisingly, even in those recipients in which direct neurorrhaphy was not possible, sensation recovery in all trigeminal territories appears. Whenever feasible, it is advocated by all teams to perform sensitive nerve neurorrhaphy. However, some patients present with complete destruction of recipient's nerves making nerve reparation impossible. This patient population do recover sensation, although a slower path of neurotisation is expected.

15.5   Survival and Complications

Current survival rate accounts for 89.3 %. Three out of 28 recipients have died by direct complications from their face transplantation. Worth noting, only one patient has died in the early postoperative period. Patient number 4 (Paris, France) died few days after a face transplant and simultaneous double hand transplantation due to sepsis and a cardiac arrest during a salvage operation. This experience depicts the difficulties that teams may experience when major VCA procedures are planned. Transplanting a large amount of composite tissues augments the risks for infectious and immunosuppression complications; thus, transplant surgeons should consider on a case-by-case scenario the indication for a simultaneous limb and face procedure. Furthermore, a good preoperative check-up for multiple resistant organisms that include real-time PCR is necessary to rule out such infections that may complicate the postoperative course with life-threatening conditions. Furthermore, patient number 4 taught surgeons another important lesson. Burn patients may be colonised by different strains of microorganisms, such as MRSA, and other multiple resistant bacteria. This theoretical colonisation put them at risk for the development of postoperative infection and sepsis. Therefore, all burn patients that are considered for VCA procedures should be examined and protected against multiple resistant bacteria infections. Burn patients have received during their hospital course large amounts of blood products and may have been treated with skin homografts. Consequently, burn survivors may have been sensitised against the HLA antigens. Crossing the major histocompatibility complex may induce acquired alloantibodies making somehow difficult correct tissue typing. Severe rejection episodes shall be expected in this situation.

Deaths of patient number 2 (China) and patient number 10 (Valencia) teach us another important lesson: patient selection. Patient number 2 died after stopping his immunosuppressant medication and implementation of alternative medicine. Patient number 10 died approximately 4 years after his face VCA by complications of his premorbid conditions (postoncological and radiotherapy deformity). Good selection and excellent team approach are a must in VCA. The risks and possible complications that this type of transplantation carries with in addition to the immunosuppression complications and side effects common to transplantation medicine make patient compliance and psychological stability absolutely necessary.

Similarly to SOT, VCA recipients may experience different types of complications and side effects from the immunosuppressant regime. So far, complications include hip necrosis, lymphoma, endometrial dysplasia, opportunistic viral infections, VCA reactivations or de novo infections, hypertension, renal failure and hyperglycaemia. Nevertheless, despite the intense immunosuppressant regimen that is commonly used in this type of transplants, good outcomes are observed with few complications. All but one patient have returned to normal life.

15.5.1   Immunological Aspects

Allograft rejection is a serious issue in organ transplantation. Skin and mucosa are well known to have a high immunogenic capacity; thus, VCA allograft rejection is always expected to be particularly intense and problematic. Acute rejection is reported in the VCA population (hand, face and other composite tissues) to be as high as 85 %, although most of the patients experience only one rejection episode. Chronic rejection, normally estimated somehow between 30 and 50 % at 5 years, has not been proven so far. However, the longest survival in face VCA is 8 years, and patients should be still followed and checked for signs of chronic rejection. All teams follow similar immunosuppressant regime: an induction therapy with corticoids and some type of lymphocyte-depleting agent (polyclonal antithymocyte globulin (ATG), anti-interleukin 2

receptor monoclonal antibodies such as daclizumab and basiliximab) and a three-drug maintenance regime (calcineurin inhibitor, steroids and mycophenolate mofetil). Some groups have developed programmes for immune tolerance with bone marrow infusion and cell therapy with diverse effects. Rejection episodes are corticoid sensitive in the majority of cases. They normally resolve with boluses of prednisone with quick taper. Some teams have utilised lymphocyte-depleting agents, but this type of treatment has some important implications for the immune and infectious disease homeostasis. Patients that receive such treatments require good antifungal and viral prophylaxis and surveillance.

15.6   Psychological Outcome

Despite the initial intense debate and the fears for potential psychological distress and identity crisis, the overall experience is extremely positive.

Several reports indicate that patients show excellent psychological outcomes. Recipients express a rapid acceptance of their new face appearance accompanied by good and quick social reintegration. Quantitative psychological tests find improvement in quality of life and physical and mental health based on the MOS-SF 12. Other tests such as SF-36 and DAS-59 produced similar results, with patients returning to work-related activities and correct social reintegration.

In fact, patients affected of severe face deformities value the procedure and risks and benefits in terms of function recovery and social reintegration. When all these items are well regained and patients may return to their premorbid life condition, a significant improvement in quality of life offsets the risks and side effects of immunosuppression and all possible complications.

Our first face transplant patient integrated quickly his new appearance (as soon as day 7, the patient was able to see and inspect his new appearance) with good psychological effects (see Figs. 15.1 and 15.2). During the first months after

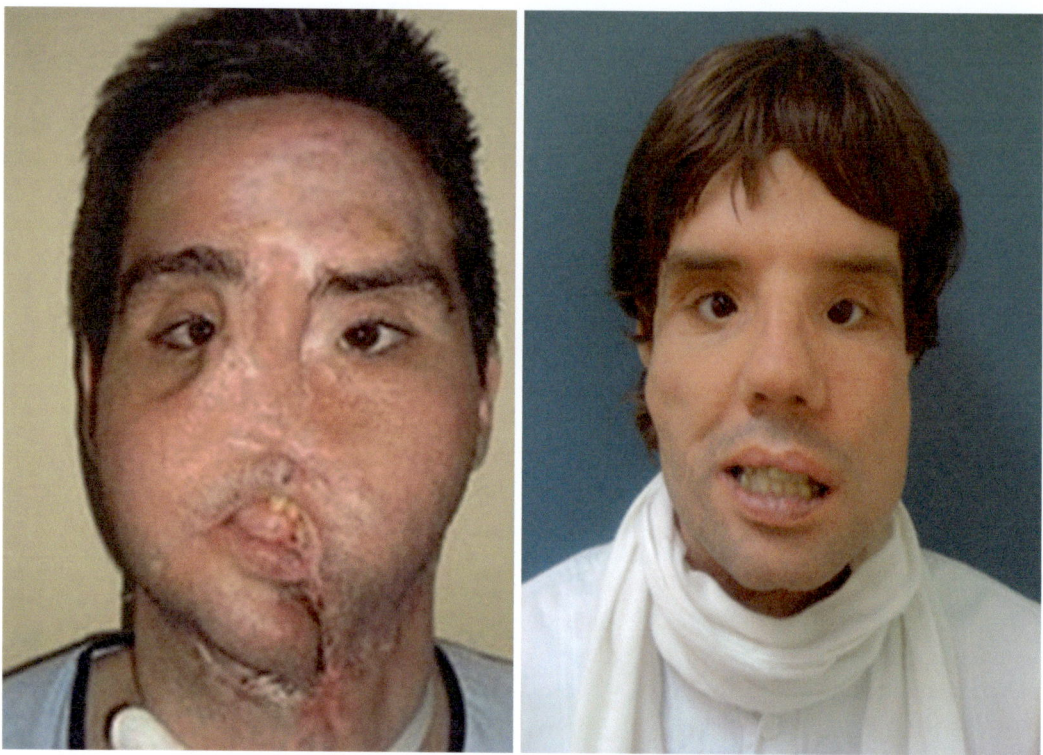

Fig. 15.1   Pre- and postoperative appearance (at 3 years) of patient number 12, Barcelona team (full-face transplant)

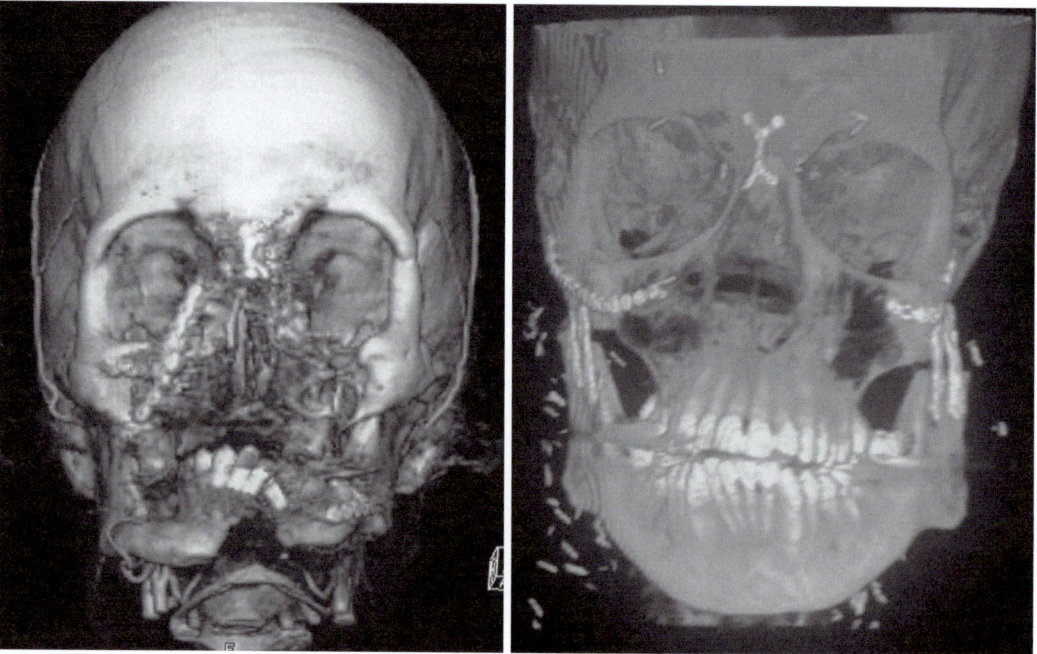

Fig. 15.2   Pre- (*left*) and postoperative (*right*) view of skeletal reconstruction (transplantation of upper and lower maxillary bone, nasal bones, palate, zygomas and teeth)

his transplant, the patient valued his experience as a significant improvement in quality of life, being worth accepting all risks and side effects. Long-term outcome has provided with the strong evidence that a robust team approach and good indication for face transplantation produce excellent functional results and correct social reintegration. Significant improvement of quality of life may offset the risks and side effects of immunosuppression, although further and longer follow-up is still necessary to define the real role of face transplantation in face reconstructive surgery.

Selected Bibliographic References

Agaoglu G, Carnevale KA, Zins JE, Siemionow M. Bilateral vascularized femoral bone transplant: a new model of vascularized bone marrow transplantation in rats, part I. Ann Plast Surg. 2006;56:658–64.

Ahern AT, Artruc SB, DellaPelle P, et al. Hyperacute rejection of HLA-AB- identical renal allografts associated with B lymphocyte and endothelial reactive antibodies. Transplantation. 1982;33:103–6.

Alam DS, Papay F, Djohan R, et al. The technical and anatomical aspects of the world's first near-total human face and maxilla transplant. Arch Face Plast Surg. 2009;11:369–77.

Altuntas SH, Zor F, Siemionow M. Total osteocutaneous hemiface allotransplantation model in rats. Plast Reconstr Surg. 2010;6S:117.

Armati PJ, Pollard JD, Gatenby P. Rat and human Schwann cells in vitro can synthesize and express MHC molecules. Muscle Nerve. 1990;13:106–16.

Arno A, Barret JP, Harrison RA, et al. Face allotransplantation and burns: a review. J Burn Care Res. 2012;33:561–76.

Arslan E, Klimczak A, Siemionow M. Chimerism induction in vascularized bone marrow transplants augmented with bone marrow cells. Microsurgery. 2007;27:190–9.

Audolfsson T, Rodríguez-Lorenzo A, Wong C, et al. Nerve transfers for face transplantation: a cadaveric study for motor and sensory restoration. Plast Reconstr Surg. 2013;131:1231–40.

Baccarani A, Follmar KE, Erdmann D, et al. Face transplantation surgical options and open problems in cadaveric models: a review article. Microsurgery. 2013;33: 239–46.

Banks ND, Hui-Chou HG, Tripathi S, et al. An anatomical study of external carotid artery vascular territories in face and midface flaps for transplantation. Plast Reconstr Surg. 2009;123:1677–87.

Barratt-Boyes SM, Thomson AW. Dendritic cells: tools and targets for transplant tolerance. Am J Transplant. 2005;5:2807–13.

Barret JP. From partial to full-face transplantation: total ablation and restoration, a change in the reconstructive paradigm. Int J Surg. 2013. doi:10.1016/j.ijsu.2013.11.016.

Barret JP, Serracanta J. LeFort I osteotomy and secondary procedures in full-face transplant patients. J Plast Reconstr Aesthet Surg. 2013;66:723–5.

Barret JP, Serracanta J, Collado JM, et al. Full face transplantation organization, development, and results–the Barcelona experience: a case report. Transplant Proc. 2011a;43:3533–4.

Barret JP, Gavaldà J, Bueno J, et al. Full face transplant: the first case report. Ann Surg. 2011b;254:252–6.

Bashour M. History and current concepts in the analysis of face attractiveness. Plast Reconstr Surg. 2006;118: 741–56.

Baumel JJ. Trigeminal-face nerve communications. Their function in face muscle innervation and reinnervation. Arch Otolaryngol. 1974;99:34–44.

Baxter-Lowe LA, Hurley CK. Advancement and clinical implications of HLA typing in allogeneic hematopoietic stem cell transplantation. Cancer Treat Res. 2009;144:1–24.

Bell-Krotoski J, Tomancik E. The repeatability of testing with Semmes-Weinstein monofilaments. J Hand Surg Am. 1987;12:155–61.

Bernard S. Microsurgical aspects of face transplantation, chapter 35. In: Siemionow MZ, editor. The know-how of face transplantation. London/New York: Springer; 2011.

Birchall M. Tongue transplantation. Lancet. 2004;363: 1663.

Black AP, Ardern-Jones MR, Kasprowicz V, et al. Human keratinocyte induction of rapid effector function in antigenspecific memory CD4+ and CD8+ T cells. Eur J Immunol. 2007;37:1485–93.

Blondeel PN, Demuynck M, Mete D, et al. Sensory nerve repair in perforator flaps for autologous breast reconstruction: sensational or senseless? Br J Plast Surg. 1999;52:37–44.

Bojovic B, Dorafshar AH, Brown EN, et al. Total face, double jaw, and tongue transplant research procurement: an educational model. Plast Reconstr Surg. 2012;130:824–34.

Borah GL, Rankin MK. Appearance is a function of the face. Plast Reconstr Surg. 2010;125:873–8.

Bos JD. Skin immune system (SIS). 2nd ed. Boca Raton/New York: CRC; 1997.

Bos JD, Kapsenberg ML. The skin immune system: progress in cutaneous biology. Immunol Today. 1993; 14:75–8.

J.P. Barret, V. Tomasello, *Face Transplantation: Principles, Techniques and Artistry*,
DOI 10.1007/978-3-662-45444-2, © Springer-Verlag Berlin Heidelberg 2015

Bos JD, Zonneveld I, Das PK, et al. The skin immune system (SIS): distribution and immunophenotype of lymphocyte subpopulations in normal human skin. J Invest Dermatol. 1987;88:569–73.

Boyd B, Mulholland S, Gullane P, et al. Reinnervated lateral antebrachial cutaneous neurosome flaps in oral reconstruction: are we making sense? Plast Reconstr Surg. 1994;93:13501359; discussion 1360–1362.

Bozkurt M, Kulahci Y, Nasir S, Klimczak A, Siemionow M. Long term survival of composite hemiface/mandible/tongue tissue allograft permitted by donor specific chimerism. Plast Reconstr Surg. 2007;120(1 Suppl):82.

Bradbury E. Understanding the problems. In: Lansdown R, Rumsey N, Bradbury E, Carr A, Partridge J, editors. Visibly different: coping with disfigurement. London: ButterworthHeineman; 1997.

Brandacher G. Composite tissue transplantation. Methods Mol Biol. 2013;1034:103–15.

Brazio PS, Barth RN, Bojovic B, et al. Algorithm for total face and multiorgan procurement from a brain-dead donor. Am J Transplant. 2013;13:2743–9.

Brown BC, McKenna SP, Siddhi K, et al. The hidden cost of skin scars: quality of life after skin scarring. J Plast Reconstr Aesthet Surg. 2008;61:1049–58.

Brown EN, Dorafshar AH, Bojovic B, et al. Total face, double jaw, and tongue transplant simulation: a cadaveric study using computer-assisted techniques. Plast Reconstr Surg. 2012;130:815–23.

Bueno J, Barret JP, Serracanta J, et al. Logistics and strategy of multiorgan procurement involving total face allograft. Am J Transplant. 2011;11:1091–7.

Bueno EM, Diaz-Siso JR, Sisk GC, et al. Vascularized composite allotransplantation and tissue engineering. J Craniofac Surg. 2013;24:256–63.

Burkat CN, Lemke BN. Anatomy of the orbit and its related structures. Otolaryngol Clin North Am. 2005; 38:825–56.

Butler PEM, Clarke A, Ashcroft R. Face transplantation: when and for whom? Am J Bioeth. 2004;4:16–7.

Butler PE, Clarke A, Hettiaratchy S. Face transplantation. BMJ. 2005;331:1349–50.

Calne RY. Prope tolerance–the future of organ transplantation from the laboratory to the clinic. Int Immunopharmacol. 2005;5:163–7.

Campana WM, Li X, Shubayev VI, Angert M, Cai K, Myers RR. Erythropoietin reduces Schwann cell TNFalpha, Wallerian degeneration and pain-related behaviors after peripheral nerve injury. Eur J Neurosci. 2006;23:617–26.

Carosella ED, Moreau P, Aractingi S, Rouas-Freiss N. HLA-G: a shield against inflammatory aggression. Trends Immunol. 2001;22:553–5.

Carroll D. A quantitative test of upper extremity function. J Chronic Dis. 1965;18:479–91.

Carty MJ, Bueno EM, Lehmann LS, et al. A position paper in support of face transplantation in the blind. Plast Reconstr Surg. 2012;130:319–24.

Carty MJ, Hivelin M, Dumontier C, et al. Lessons learned from simultaneous face and bilateral hand allotransplantation. Plast Reconstr Surg. 2013;132:423–32.

Caterson EJ, Diaz-Siso JR, Shetye P, et al. Craniofacial principles in face transplantation. J Craniofac Surg. 2012;23:1234–8.

Cavadas PC, Ibáñez J, Thione A. Surgical aspects of a lower face, mandible, and tongue allotransplantation. J Reconstr Microsurg. 2012;28:43–7.

Cendales LC, Kanittakis J, Schneeberger N, et al. The Banff 2007 working classification of skin-containing composite tissue allograft pathology. Am J Transplant. 2008;8:1396–400.

Chandawarkar AA, Diaz-Siso JR, Bueno EM, et al. Face appearance transfer and persistence after three-dimensional virtual face transplantation. Plast Reconstr Surg. 2013;132:957–66.

Chang G, Pomahac B. Psychosocial changes 6 months after face transplantation. Psychosomatics. 2013;54:367–71.

Cheng K, Zhou S, Jiang K, et al. Microsurgical replantation of the avulsed scalp: report of 20 cases. Plast Reconstr Surg. 1996;97(6):1099–106.

Clarke A, Butler PE. Face transplantation: adding to the reconstructive options after severe face injury and disease. Expert Opin Biol Ther. 2005;5:1539–46.

Coffman KL, Siemionow MZ. Face transplantation: psychological outcomes at three-year follow-up. Psychosomatics. 2013;54:372–8.

Coleman SR. Face augmentation with structural fat grafting. Clin Plast Surg. 2006;33:567–77.

Constable AL, Armati PJ, Toyka KV, Hartung HP. Production of prostanoids by Lewis rat Schwann cells in vitro. Brain Res. 1994;635:75–80.

Cutler CW, Jotwani R. Dendritic cells at the oral mucosal interface. J Dent Res. 2006;85:678–89.

Dellon AL, Andonian E, DeJesus RA. Measuring sensibility of the trigeminal nerve. Plast Reconstr Surg. 2007;120:1546–50.

Demir Y, Ozmen S, Klimczak A, et al. Tolerance induction in composite face allograft transplantation in the rat model. Plast Reconstr Surg. 2004;114:1790–801.

Devauchelle B, Badet L, Lengele B, et al. First human face allograft: early report. Lancet. 2006;368:203–9.

Diaz-Siso JR, Bueno EM, Sisk GC, et al. Vascularized composite tissue allotransplantation–state of the art. Clin Transplant. 2013a;27:330–7.

Diaz-Siso JR, Parker M, Bueno EM, et al. Face allotransplantation: a 3-year follow-up report. J Plast Reconstr Aesthet Surg. 2013b;66:1458–63.

Dodson TB, Kaban LB. Recommendations for management of trigeminal nerve defects based on a critical appraisal of the literature. J Oral Maxillofac Surg. 1997;55:1380–6; discussion 1387.

Dorafshar AH, Bojovic B, Christy MR, et al. Total face, double jaw, and tongue transplantation: an evolutionary concept. Plast Reconstr Surg. 2013;13:241–51.

Dubernard JM. Hand and face allografts: myth, dream, and reality. Proc Am Philos Soc. 2011;155:13–22.

Dubernard JM, Devauchelle B. Face transplantation. Lancet. 2008;372:603–4.

Dubernard JM, Own E, Herberg G, et al. Human hand allograft: report on first 6 months. Lancet. 1999;353: 1315–20.

Dubernard JM, Lengele B, Morelon E, et al. Outcomes 18 months after the first human partial face transplantation. N Engl J Med. 2007;357:2451–60.

Edrich T, Cywinski JB, Colomina MJ, et al. Perioperative management of face transplantation: a survey. Anesth Analg. 2012;115:668–70.

Eduardo Bermudez L, Santamaria A, Romero T, et al. Experimental model of face transplant. Plast Reconstr Surg. 2002;110:1374–5.

Einecke G, Sis B, Reeve J, et al. Antibody-mediated microcirculation injury is the major cause of late Kidney transplant failure. Am J Transplant. 2009;9: 2520–31.

Essick GK, Phillips C, Kim SH, et al. Sensory retraining following orthognathic surgery: effect on threshold measures of sensory function. J Oral Rehabil. 2009;36: 415–26.

Follmar KE, Baccarani A, Das RR, et al. Osteocutaneous face transplantation. J Plast Reconstr Aesthet Surg. 2008;61:518–24.

Friedman JM. Neurofibromatosis 1. In: Pagon RA, Bird TD, Dolan CR, et al., editors. Gene reviews. Seattle: University of Washington; 1993.

Fung J, Kelly D, Kadry Z, Patel-Tom K, Eghtesad B. Immunosuppression in liver transplantation: beyond calcineurin inhibitors. Liver Transpl. 2005;11: 267–80.

Furnas DW. The retaining ligaments of the cheek. Plast Reconstr Surg. 1989;83:11–6.

Gharb BB, Rampazzo A, Siemionow MZ. The sensory recovery in face transplantation. Capitolo 16. In: Siemionow MZ, editor. The know-how of face transplantation. London/New York: Springer; 2011.

Gharb BB, Rampazzo A, Altuntas SH, et al. Effectiveness of topical immunosuppressants in prevention and treatment of rejection in face allotransplantation. Transplantation. 2013;95:1197–203.

Girnita AL, McCurry KR, Zeevi A. Increased lung allograft failure in patients with HLA-specific antibody. Clin Transpl. 2007;231–239.

Gold BG. FK506 and the role of the immunophilin FKBP-52 in nerve regeneration. Drug Metab Rev. 1999;31: 649–63.

Gomez-Cia T, Infante-Cossio P, Sicilia-castro D, et al. Sequence of multiorgan procurement involving face allograft. Am J Transplant. 2011a;11:2261.

Gomez-Cia T, Sicilia-castro D, Infante-Cossio P, et al. Second human face allotransplantation to restore a severe defect following radical resection of bilateral massive plexiform neurofibromas. Plast Reconstr Surg. 2011b;127:995–6.

Gordon CR, Siemionow M. Requirements for the development of a hand transplantation program. Ann Plast Surg. 2009;63:262–73.

Gordon CR, Tai CY, Suzuki H, et al. Review of vascularized bone marrow transplantation: current status and future clinical applications. Microsurgery. 2007;27:348–53.

Gordon CR, Siemionow M, Papay F, et al. The world's experience with face transplantation. What have we learned thus far? Ann Plast Surg. 2009;63:572–8.

Gottlieb L, Agarwal S. Autologous alternatives to face transplantation. J Reconstr Microsurg. 2012;28:49–61.

Gozel-Ulusal B, Ulusal AE, Ozmen S, et al. A new composite face and scalp transplantation model in the rat. Plast Reconstr Surg. 2003;112:1302–11.

Grant GA, Goodkin R, Kliot M. Evaluation and surgical management of peripheral nerve problems. Neurosurgery. 1999;44:825–39; discussion 39–40.

Greaves MW. Physiology of skin. J Invest Dermatol. 1976;67:66–9.

Greek R, Pippus A, Hansen LA. The Nuremberg Code subverts human health and safety by requiring animal modeling. BMC Med Ethics. 2012;13:16.

Gribbin J, Gribbin M. Being human. London: Phoenix; 1995.

Grone A. Keratinocytes and cytokines. Vet Immunol Immunopathol. 2002;88:1–12.

Guimberteau JC, Baudet I, Panconi B, et al. Human allotransplant of a digital flexion system ascularized on the ulnar pedicle: a preliminary report and 1-year follow up of two cases. Plast Reconstr Surg. 1992;89:1135–47.

Guo S, Han Y, Zhang X, et al. Human face allotransplantation: a 2-year follow-up study. Lancet. 2008;372:631–8.

Han DG. Pain around the ear in bell's palsy is referred pain of face nerve origin: the role of nervi nervorum. Med Hypotheses. 2010;74:235–6.

Hanmugarajah K, Hettiaratchy S, Butler PE. Face transplantation. Curr Opin Otolaryngol Head Neck Surg. 2012;20:291–7.

Hauner H, Loffler G. Adipose tissue development: the role of precursor cells and adipogenic factors. Part I: adipose tissue development and the role of precursor cells. Klin Wochenschr. 1987;65:803–11.

Hausman GJ. Adipocyte development in subcutaneous tissues of the young rat. Acta Anat (Basel). 1982;112: 185–96.

Hausman GJ, Campion DR, McNamara JP, Richardson RL, Martin RJ. Adipose tissue development in the fetal pig after decapitation. J Anim Sci. 1981;53:1634–44.

Heeger PS, Dinavahi R. Transplant immunology for non-immunologist. Mt Sinai J Med. 2012;79:376–87.

Henri S, Siret C, Machy P, et al. Mature DC from skin and skin-draining LN retain the ability to acquire and efficiently present targeted antigen. Eur J Immunol. 2007;37:1184–93.

Hequet O, Morelon E, Bourgeot JP, et al. Allogeneic donor bone marrow cells recovery and infusion after allogeneic face transplantation from the same donor. Bone Marrow Transplant. 2008;41:1059–61.

Hermanson A, Dalsgaard CJ, Arnander C, et al. Sensibility and cutaneous reinnervation in free flaps. Plast Reconstr Surg. 1987;79:422–7.

Hettiaratchy S, Butler PE. Face transplantation – fantasy or the future? Lancet. 2002;360:56.

Hettiaratchy S, Randolph MA, Petit F, et al. Composite tissue allotransplantation—a new era in plastic surgery? Br J Plast Surg. 2004;57:381–91.

Hivelin M, Siemionow M, Grimbert P, et al. Extracorporeal photopheresis: from solid organs to face transplantation. Transpl Immunol. 2009;21:117–28.

Hofmann GO, Kirschner MH, Wagner FD, et al. Allogeneic vascularized transplantation of human femoral diaphyses and total knee joints—first clinical experiences. Transplant Proc. 1998;30:2754–61.

Honn M, Go G. The ideal of face beauty: a review. J Orofac Orthop. 2007;68:6–16.

Hornung DE. Nasal anatomy and the sense of smell. Adv Otorhinolaryngol. 2006;63:1–22.

Horta R, Monteiro D, Valença-Filipe R, et al. Face allotransplantation procurement using a transparotid approach: a new anatomical model. Microsurgery. 2013. doi:10.1002/micr.22216.

Houseman ND, Taylor GI, Pan WR. The angiosomes of the head and neck: anatomic study and clinical applications. Plast Reconstr Surg. 2000;105:2287–313.

Hu W, Lu J, Zhang L, et al. A preliminary report of penile transplantation. Eur Urol. 2006;50:851–3.

Hui-Chou HG, Nam AJ, Rodriguez ED. Clinical face composite tissue allotransplantation: a review of the first four global experiences and future implications. Plast Reconstr Surg. 2010;125:538–46.

Infante-Cossio P, Barrera-Pulido F, Gomez-Cia T, et al. Face transplantation: a concise update. Med Oral Patol Oral Cir Bucal. 2013;18:e263–71.

Jameson J, Havran WL. Skin gammadelta T-cell functions in homeostasis and wound healing. Immunol Rev. 2007;215:114–22.

Jelks GW, Jelks EB. The influence of orbital and eyelid anatomy on the palpebral aperture. Clin Plast Surg. 1991;18:183–95.

Jesitus J. Chinese transplant surgery. Cosmet Surg Times. 2006;9:12–4.

Jones TR, Humphrey PA, Brennan DC. Transplantation of vascularized allogeneic skeletal muscle for scalp reconstruction in renal transplant patient. Transplant Proc. 1998;30:2746–53.

Jones JW, Ustuner T, Zdichavscky M, et al. Long-term survival of an extremity composite tissue allograft with FK506-mycophenolate mofetil therapy. Surgery. 1999;126:384–8.

Jones JW, Gruber SA, Barker JH, Breidenbach WC. Successful hand transplantation. One-year follow-up. Louisville Hand transplant team. N Engl J Med. 2000;343:468–73.

Jotwani R, Cutler CW. Multiple dendritic cell (DC) subpopulations in human gingiva and association of mature DCs with CD4+ T-cells in situ. J Dent Res. 2003;82:736–41.

Jotwani R, Palucka AK, Al-Quotub M, et al. Mature dendritic cells infiltrate the T cell-rich region of oral mucosa in chronic periodontitis: in situ, in vivo, and in vitro studies. J Immunol. 2001;167:4693–700.

Kanitakis J, Cendales LC. Classification of face rejection: Banff classification for CTA, capitolo 18. In: Siemionow MZ, editor. The know-how of face transplantation. London/New York: Springer; 2011.

Kaufman CL, Ouseph R, Marvin MR, et al. Monitoring and long-term outcomes in vascularized composite allotransplantation. Curr Opin Organ Transplant. 2013;18:652–8.

Kawai T, Cosimi AB, Spitzer TR, et al. HLA-mismatched renal transplantation without maintenance immunosuppression. N Engl J Med. 2008;358:353–61.

Kerawala CJ, Newlands C, Martin I. Spontaneous sensory recovery in non- innervated radial forearm flaps used for head and neck reconstruction. Int J Oral Maxillofac Surg. 2006;35:714–7.

Kiefer R, Kieseier BC, Stoll G, Hartung HP. The role of macrophages in immune- mediated damage to the peripheral nervous system. Prog Neurobiol. 2001;64:109–27.

Kieseier BC, Hartung HP, Wiendl H. Immune circuitry in the peripheral nervous system. Curr Opin Neurol. 2006;19:437–45.

Kiwanuka H, Bueno EM, Diaz-Siso JR, et al. Evolution of ethical debate on face transplantation. Plast Reconstr Surg. 2013;132:1558–68.

Klimczak A, Siemionow M. Immunology of tissue transplantation. In: Siemionow M, Eisenmann-Klein M, editors. Plastic and reconstructive surgery. London: Springer; 2010.

Kulahci Y, Siemionow M. A new composite hemiface/mandible/tongue transplantation model in rats. Ann Plast Surg. 2010;64:114–21.

Kulahci Y, Klimczak A, Siemionow M. Long term survival of composite hemiface/mandible/tongue tissue allograft permitted by donor specific chimerism. Plast Reconst Surg. 2006;118(4 Suppl):34.

Lahteenmaki T, Waris T, Asko-Seljavaara S, et al. The return of sensitivity to cold, warmth and pain from excessive heat in free microvascular flaps. Scand J Plast Reconstr Surg Hand Surg. 1991;25:143–50.

Lamparello BM, Bueno EM, Diaz-Siso JR, et al. Face time: educating face transplant candidates. Eplasty. 2013;13:e36.

Langlois JH, Kalakanis L, Rubenstein AJ, et al. Maxims or myths of beauty? A metaanalytic and theoretical review. Psychol Bull. 2000;126:390–423.

Lantieri L. Face transplant: a paradigm change in face reconstruction. J Craniofac Surg. 2012;23:250–3.

Lantieri L, Meningaud JP, Grimbert P, et al. Repair of the lower and middle parts of the face by composite tissue allotransplantation in a patient with massive plexiform neurofibroma: a 1-year follow-up study. Lancet. 2008;372:639–45.

Lantieri L, Hivelin M, Audard V, et al. Feasibility, reproducibility, risks and benefits of face transplantation: a prospective study of outcomes. Am J Transplant. 2011;11:367–78.

Lanzetta M, Petruzzo P, Dubernard JM, et al. Second report (1998–2006) of the International Registry of Hand and Composite Tissue Transplantation. Transpl Immunol. 2007;18:1–6.

Lengele B. Current concepts and future challenges in face transplantation. Clin Plast Surg. 2009;36:507–21.

Leonard DA, Gordon CR, Sachs DH, et al. Immunobiology of face transplantation. J Craniofac Surg. 2012;23: 268–71.

Leonard DA, Cetrulo Jr CL, McGrouther DA, et al. Induction of tolerance of vascularized composite allografts. Transplantation. 2013;95:403–9.

Leto Barone AA, Sun Z, Montgomery RA, et al. Impact of donor-specific antibodies in reconstructive transplantation. Expert Rev Clin Immunol. 2013;9:835–44.

Levi DM, Tzakis AG, Kato T, et al. Transplantation of the abdominal wall. Lancet. 2003;361:2173–6.

Lierde KM, Roche N, Letter MD, et al. Speech characteristics one year after first Belgian face transplantation. Laryngoscope. 2014. doi:10.1002/lary.24585.

Liu YJ. IPC: professional type 1 interferon-producing cells and plasmacytoid dendritic cell precursors. Annu Rev Immunol. 2005;23:275–306.

Loffler G, Hauner H. Adipose tissue development: the role of precursor cells and adipogenic factors. Part II: the regulation of the adipogenic conversion by hormones and serum factors. Klin Wochenschr. 1987;65:812–7.

Losee JE, Fletcher DR, Gorantla VS. Human face allotransplantation: patient selection and pertinent considerations. J Craniofac Surg. 2012;23:260–4.

Ma W, Pober JS. Human endothelial cells effectively costimulate cytokine production by, but not differentiation of, naïve CD4+ T cells. J Immunol. 1998;161:2158–67.

Mackinnon SE, Doolabh VB, Novak CB, et al. Clinical outcome following nerve allograft transplantation. Plast Reconstr Surg. 2001;107:1419–29.

Martinez-Madrigal F, Micheau C. Histology of the major salivary glands. Am J Surg Pathol. 1989;13:879–99.

Mathers AR, Larregina AT. Professional antigen-presenting cells of the skin. Immunol Res. 2006;36:127–36.

McDonald CJ. Structure and function of the skin. Are there differences between black and white skin? Dermatol Clin. 1988;6:343–7.

Meningaud JP, Paraskevas A, Ingallina F, et al. Face transplant graft procurement: a preclinical and clinical study. Plast Reconstr Surg. 2008;122:1383–9.

Meningaud JP, Benjoar MD, Hivelin M, et al. The procurement of total human face graft for allotransplantation: a preclinical Study and the first clinical case. Plast Reconstr Surg. 2010;126:1181–90.

Meningaud JP, Hivelin M, Benjoar MD, et al. The procurement of allotransplants for ballistic trauma: a preclinical study and a report of two clinical cases. Plast Reconstr Surg. 2011;127:1892–900.

Meyer ZU, Horste G, Hu W, et al. The immunocompetence of Schwann cells. Muscle Nerve. 2008;37:3–13.

Monaco AP. Prospects and strategies for clinical tolerance. Transplant Proc. 2004a;36:227–31.

Monaco AP. The beginning of clinical tolerance in solid organ allografts. Exp Clin Transplant. 2004b;2:153–61.

Morales-Buenrostro LE, Castro R, Terasaki PI. A single human leukocyte antigen- antibody test after heart or lung transplantation is predictive of survival. Transplantation. 2008;85:478–81.

Morris P, Bradley A, Doyal L, et al. Face transplantation: a review of the technical, immunological, psychological and clinical issues with recommendations for good practice. Transplantation. 2007;83:109–28.

Murase N, Starzl TE, Tanabe M, et al. Variable chimerism, graft-versushost disease, and tolerance after different kinds of cell and whole organ transplantation from Lewis to brown Norway rats. Transplantation. 1995;60:158–71.

Murphy BD, Zuker RM, Borschel GH. Vascularized composite allotransplantation: an update on medical and surgical progress and remaining challenges. J Plast Reconstr Aesthet Surg. 2013;66:1449–55.

Mutyambizi K, Berger CL, Edelson RL. The balance between immunity and tolerance: the role of Langerhans cells. Cell Mol Life Sci. 2009;66:831–40.

Nagaraju K, Raben N, Merritt G, Loeffler L, Kirk K, Plotz P. A variety of cytokines and immunologically relevant surface molecules are expressed by normal human skeletal muscle cells under proinflammatory stimuli. Clin Exp Immunol. 1998;113:407–14.

Neskey D, Eloy JA, Casiano RR. Nasal, septal, and turbinate anatomy and embryology. Otolaryngol Clin North Am. 2009;42:193–205.

O'Sullivan NL, Skandera CA, Montgomery PC. Lymphocyte lineages at mucosal effector sites: rat salivary glands. J Immunol. 2001;166:5522–9.

Okie S. Brave new face. Face transplantation. N Engl J Med. 2006;354:889–94.

Opelz G. New immunosuppressants and HLA matching. Transplant Proc. 2001;33:467–8.

Opelz G. Non-HLA transplantation immunity revealed by lymphocytotoxic antibodies. Lancet. 2005;365:1570–6.

Ozer K, Gurunluoglu R, Zielinski M, et al. Extension of composite tissue allograft survival across major histocompatibility barrier under short course of antilymphocyte serum and cyclosporine a therapy. J Reconstr Microsurg. 2003a;19:249–56.

Ozer K, Oke R, Gurunluoglu R, et al. Induction of tolerance to hind limb allografts in rats receiving cyclosporine A and antilymphocyte serum: effect of duration of the treatment. Transplantation. 2003b;75:31–6.

Ozmen S, Ulusal BG, Ulusal AE, et al. Composite vascularized skin/bone transplantation models for bone marrow-based tolerance studies. Ann Plast Surg. 2006;56:295–300.

Ozmen S, Findikcioglu F, Sezgin B, et al. Would you be a face transplant donor? A survey of the Turkish population about face allotransplantation. Ann Plast Surg. 2013;71:233–7.

Perry SS, Kim M, Spangrude GJ. Direct effects of cyclosporin A on proliferation of hematopoietic stem and progenitor cells. Cell Transplant. 1999;8:339–44.

Petit F, Paraskevas A, Minns AB, et al. Face transplantation: where do we stand? Plast Reconstr Surg. 2004a;113:1429–33.

Petit F, Paraskevas A, Lantieri L. A surgeons' perspective on the ethics of face transplantation. Am J Bioeth. 2004b;4:14–6.

Petruzzo P, Lanzetta M, Dubernard JM, et al. The international Registry on hand and composite tissue transplantation. Transplantation. 2008;86:487–92.

Petruzzo P, Kanitakis J, Badet L, et al. Long-term follow-up in composite tissue allotransplantation: in-depth study of five (hand and face) recipients. Am J Transplant. 2011;11:808–16.

Petruzzo P, Testelin S, Kanitakis J, et al. First human face transplantation: 5 years outcomes. Transplantation. 2012;93:236–40.

Pirnay P, Foo R, Hervé C, et al. Ethical questions raised by the first allotransplantations of the face: a survey of French surgeons. J Craniomaxillofac Surg. 2012;40: e402–7.

Place MJ, Song T, Hardesty RA, et al. Sensory reinnervation of autologous tissue TRAM flaps after breast reconstruction. Ann Plast Surg. 1997;38:19–22.

Pomahac B. Establishing a composite tissue allotransplantation program. J Reconstr Microsurg. 2012; 28:3–6.

Pomahac B, Pribaz J. Face composite tissue allograft. J Craniofac Surg. 2012;23:265–7.

Pomahac B, Lengele B, Ridgway EB, et al. Vascular considerations in composite midfacial allotransplantation. Plast Reconstr Surg. 2010;125:517–22.

Pomahac B, Papay F, Bueno EM, ct al. Donor face composite allograft recovery operation: Cleveland and Boston experiences. Plast Reconstr Surg. 2012a;129: 461e–7.

Pomahac B, Pribaz J, Eriksson E, et al. Three patients with full face transplantation. N Engl J Med. 2012b; 366:715–22.

Pomahac B, Pribaz JJ, Bueno EM, et al. Novel surgical technique for full face transplantation. Plast Reconstr Surg. 2012c;130:549–55.

Pomahac B, Bueno EM, Sisk GC, et al. Current principles of face allotransplantation: the Brigham and Women's Hospital Experience. Plast Reconstr Surg. 2013;131:1069–76.

Pree I, Pilat N, Wekerle T. Recent progress in tolerance induction through mixed chimerism. Int Arch Allergy Immunol. 2007;144:254–66.

Quilichini J, Hivelin M, Benjoar MD, et al. Restoration of the donor after face graft procurement for allotransplantation: report on the technique and outcomes of seven cases. Plast Reconstr Surg. 2012;129:1105–11.

Radu CA, Horn D, Kiefer J, et al. Donor-derived transplant acceptance-inducing cells in composite tissue allotransplantation. J Plast Reconstr Aesthet Surg. 2012;65:1684–91.

Rankin M, Borah GL. Perceived functional impact of abnormal face appearance. Plast Reconstr Surg. 2003;111:2140–6.

Ren X, Laugel MC. The next frontier in composite tissue allotransplantation. CNS Neurosci Ther. 2013;19:1–4.

Robey PG, Bianco P. The use of adult stem cells in rebuilding the human face. J Am Dent Assoc. 2006;137: 961–72.

Rodriguez-Lorenzo A, Audolfsson T, Rozen S, et al. Supraorbitary to infraorbitary nerve transfer for restoration of midface sensation in face transplantation: cadaver feasibility study. Microsurgery. 2012;32:309–13.

Rüegg EM, Hivelin M, Hemery F, et al. Face transplantation program in France: a cost analysis of five patients. Transplantation. 2012;93:1166–72.

Rumsey N. Psychological aspects of face transplantation: read the small print carefully. Am J Bioeth. 2004;4:22–5.

Rumsey N, Harcourt D. Body image and disfigurement: issues and interventions. Body Image. 2004;1:83–97.

Rumsey N, Harcourt D. Visible difference amongst children and adolescents: issues and interventions. Dev Neurorehabil. 2007;10:113–23.

Rumsey N, Clarke A, White P, et al. Altered body image: appearance-related concerns of people with visible disfigurement. J Adv Nurs. 2004;48:443–53.

Sachs DH. Mixed chimerism as an approach to transplantation tolerance. Clin Immunol. 2000;95:S63–8.

Sahin M. Chapter 589. Neurocutaneous syndromes. In: Kliegman RM, Stanton BF, St Geme J, Schor N, Behrman RE, editors. Nelston textbook of pediatrics. 19th ed. Philadelphia: Saunders Elsevier; 2011.

Santanelli F, Tenna S, Pace A, Scuderi N. Free flap reconstruction of the sole of the foot with or without sensory nerve coaptation. Plast Reconstr Surg. 2002;109:2314–22; discussion 2323–4.

Schultes G, Gaggl A, Karcher H. Neuronal anastomosis of the cutaneous ramus of the intercostal nerve to achieve sensibility in the latissimus dorsi transplant. J Oral Maxillofac Surg. 2000;58:36–9.

Sedaghati-nia A, Gilton A, Liger C, et al. Anaesthesia and intensive care management of face transplantation. Br J Anaesth. 2013;111:600–6.

Shevach EM. Suppressor T, cells: rebirth, function and homeostasis. Curr Biol. 2000a;10:R572–5.

Shevach EM. Regulatory T, cells in autoimmmunity*. Annu Rev Immunol. 2000b;18:423–49.

Shrestha BM. The Declaration of Helsinki in relation to medical research: historical and current perspectives. J Nepal Health Res Counc. 2012;10:254–7.

Siemionow M. Impact of reconstructive transplantation on the future of plastic and reconstructive surgery. Clin Plast Surg. 2012;39:425–34.

Siemionow M, Agaoglu G. The issue of "face appearance and identity transfer" after mock transplantation: a cadaver study in preparation for face allograft transplantation in humans. J Reconstr Microsurg. 2006;22:329–34.

Siemionow M, Agaoglu G. Tissue transplantation in plastic surgery. Clin Plast Surg. 2007;34:251–69.

Siemionow M, Gordon CR. Overview of guidelines for establishing a face transplant program: a work in progress. Am J Transplant. 2010;10:1290–6.

Siemionow M, Klimczak A. Tolerance and future directions for composite tissue allograft transplants: part II. Plast Reconstr Surg. 2009;123:7e–17.

Siemionow M, Kulahci Y. Experimental models of composite tissue allograft transplants. Semin Plast Surg. 2007;21:205–12.

Siemionow MZ, Nasir S. Impact of donor bone marrow on survival of composite tissue allografts. Ann Plast Surg. 2008;60:455–62.

Siemionow M, Ozturk C. Donor operation for face transplantation. J Reconstr Microsurg. 2012a;28:35–42.

Siemionow M, Ozturk C. Face transplantation: outcomes, concerns, controversies, and future directions. J Craniofac Surg. 2012b;23:254–9.

Siemionow M, Sonmez E. Face as an organ. Ann Plast Surg. 2008;61:345–52.

Siemionow M, Yalcin K. Face transplantation. Semin Plast Surg. 2007;21:259–68.

Siemionow MZ, Zor F. Experimental studies in face transplantation: rodent model. In: Siemionow MZ, editor. The know-how of face transplantation. London/New York: Springer; 2011.

Siemionow M, Gozel-Ulusal B, Ulusal A, et al. Functional tolerance following face transplantation in the rat. Transplantation. 2003a;75:1607–9.

Siemionow MZ, Izycki DM, Zielinski M. Donor-specific tolerance in fully major histocompatibility major histocompatibility complex-mismatched limb allograft transplants under an antialphabeta T-cell receptor monoclonal antibody and cyclosporine A protocol. Transplantation. 2003b;76:1662–8.

Siemionow M, Ozmen S, Demir Y. Prospects for face allograft transplantation in humans. Plast Reconstr Surg. 2004a;113:1421–8.

Siemionow M, Ulusal BG, Ozmen S, et al. Composite vascularized skin/bone graft model: a viable source for vascularized bone marrow transplantation. Microsurgery. 2004b;24:200–6.

Siemionow M, Demir Y, Mukherjee A, et al. Development and maintenance of donor-specific chimerism in semiallogenic and fully MHC mismatched face allograft transplants. Transplantation. 2005a;79:558–67.

Siemionow MZ, Demir Y, Sari A, Klimczak A. Face tissue allograft transplantation. Transplant Proc. 2005b; 37:201–4.

Siemionow M, Papay F, Kulahci Y, et al. Coronal-posterior approach for face/scalp flap harvesting in preparation for face transplantation. J Reconstr Microsurg. 2006a; 22:399–405.

Siemionow M, Unal S, Agaoglu G, Sari A. A cadaver study in preparation for face allograft transplantation in humans: part I. What are alternative sources for total face defect coverage? Plast Reconstr Surg. 2006b;117:864–72.

Siemionow M, Agaoglu G, Unal S. A cadaver study in preparation for face allograft transplantation in humans: part II Mock face transplantation. Plast Reconstr Surg. 2006c;117:876–85.

Siemionow M, Izycki D, Ozer K, et al. Role of thymus in operational tolerance induction in limb allograft transplant model. Transplantation. 2006d;81:1568–76.

Siemionow M, Papay F, Alam D, et al. Near-total human face transplantation for a severely disfigured patient in the USA. Lancet. 2009;374:203–9.

Siemionow M, Zor F, Gordon CR. Face and upper extremity transplantation: future challenges and potential concerns. Plast Reconstr Surg. 2010a;1263:08–15.

Siemionow M, Papay F, Djohan R, et al. First U.S. near-total human face transplantation – a paradigm shift for massive face injuries. Plast Reconstr Surg. 2010b;125:111–22.

Siemionow MZ, Ozturk C, Altuntas S. An update on face transplants performed between 2005 and 2010. Capitolo 44. In: Siemionow MZ, editor. The know- how of face transplantation. London/New York: Springer; 2011a.

Siemionow M, Gatherwright J, Djoham R, et al. Cost analysis of conventional face reconstruction procedures followed by face transplantation. Am J Transplant. 2011b;11:379–85.

Siemionow M, Madajka M, Cwykiel J. Application of cell-based therapies in face transplantation. Ann Plast Surg. 2012;69:575–9.

Siemionow M, Gharb BB, Rampazzo A. Successes and lessons learned after more than a decade of upper extremity and face transplantation. Curr Opin Organ Transplant. 2013;18:633–9.

Singhal D, Pribaz JJ, Pomahac B. The Brigham and Women's Hospital face transplant program: a look back. Plast Reconstr Surg. 2012;129:89e–91.

Sisk GC, Kumamaru KK, Schultz K, et al. Cine computed tomography angiography evaluation of blood flow for full face transplant surgical planning. Eplasty. 2012; 12:e57.

Soga S, Pomahac B, Wake N, et al. CT angiography for surgical planning in face transplantation candidates. AJNR Am J Neuroradiol. 2013;34:1873–81.

Sonmez A, Bayramicli M, Sonmez B, et al. Reconstruction of the weight – bearing surface of the foot with non-neurosensory free flaps. Plast Reconstr Surg. 2003;111: 2230–6.

Sosa I, Reyes O, Kuffler DP. Immunosuppressants: neuroprotection and promoting neurological recovery following peripheral nerve and spinal cord lesions. Exp Neurol. 2005;195:7–15.

Spurgeon B. Surgeons pleased with patient's progress after face transplant. BMJ. 2005;331:1359.

Starzl TE, Demetris AJ, Murase N, et al. Cell migration, chimerism, and graft acceptance. Lancet. 1992;339: 1579–82.

Starzl TE, Demetris AJ, Trucco M, et al. Cell migration and chimerism after whole-organ transplantation: the basis of graft acceptance. Hepatology. 1993;17: 1127–52.

Stassen M, Schmitt E, Jonuleit H. Human CD(4+) CD(25+) regulatory T cells and infectious tolerance. Transplantation. 2004;77:S23–5.

Strome M, Stein I, Esclamado R, et al. Laryngeal transplantation and 40-month follow-up. N Engl J Med. 2001;344:1676–9.

Strouse TB, Wolkott DL, Skotzko CE. Transplantation. In: txtbook of consultation-liassion psychiatry. American psychiatric press, 1996.

Sulaiman OA, Voda J, Gold BG, et al. FK506 increases peripheral nerve regeneration after chronic axotomy but not after chronic Schwann cell denervation. Exp Neurol. 2002;175:127–37.

Sumpio BE, Riley JT, Dardik A. Cells in focus: endothelial cell. Int J Biochem Cell Biol. 2002;34: 1508–12.

Takamatsu A, Harashina T, Inoue T. Selection of appropriate recipient vessels in difficult, microsurgical head and neck reconstruction. J Reconstr Microsurg. 1996;12:499–507; discussion 508–13.

The first face transplant. [Editorial] Lancet 2005;366: 1984.

Thomander L, Arvidsson J, Aldskogius H. Distribution of sensory ganglion cells innervating face muscles in the cat. An anatomical study with the horseradish peroxidase technique. Acta Otolaryngol. 1982;94:81–92.

Thomas A. Total face and scalp replantation. Plast Reconstr Surg. 1998;102:2085.

Thorne CH. Face lift. In: Thorne CH, editor. Grabb and Smith's plastic surgery. Philadelphia: Wolters Kluwer Health/Lippincott Williams & Wilkins; 2007. p. 498–508.

Tindholdt TT, Tonseth KA. Spontaneous reinnervation of deep inferior epigastric artery perforator flaps after secondary breast reconstruction. Scand J Plast Reconstr Surg Hand Surg. 2008;42:28–31.

Tobin GR, Breidenbach III WC, Pidwell III DJ, et al. Transplantation of the hand, face, and composite structures: evolution and current status. Clin Plast Surg. 2007;34:271–8.

Udina E, Voda J, Gold BG, et al. Comparative dosedependence study of FK506 on transected mouse sciatic nerve repaired by allograft or xenograft. J Peripher Nerv Syst. 2003;8:145–54.

Unal S, Agaoglu G, Zins J, et al. New surgical approach in face transplantation extends survival of allograft recipients. Ann Plast Surg. 2005;55(3):297–303.

Ustuner ET. Long-term composite tissue allograft survival in a porcine model with cyclosporine/mycophenolate mofetil therapy. Transplantation. 1998;66:1581.

Ustuner ET. Swine composite tissue allotransplant model for preclinical transplant studies. Microsurgery. 2000;20:400.

Vasilic D, Alloway RR, Barker JH, et al. Risk assessment of immunosuppressive therapy in face transplantation. Plast Reconstr Surg. 2007;120:657–68.

Wang MS, Zeleny-Pooley M, Gold BG. Comparative dose dependence study of FK506 and Cyclosporine A on the rate of axonal regeneration in the rat sciatic nerve. J Pharmacol Exp Ther. 1997;282:1084–93.

Wang J, Dong Y, Sun JZ, et al. Donor lymphoid organs are a major site of alloreactive T-cell priming following intestinal transplantation. Am J Transplant. 2006;6:2563–71.

Waxman SG. The autonomic nervous system. In: Clinical neuroanatomy. New York: McGraw-Hill; 2010. p. 248–63.

Weissenbacher A, Hautz T, Pratschke J, et al. Vascularized composite allografts and solid organ transplants: similarities and differences. Curr Opin Organ Transplant. 2013;18:640–4.

Wiendl H, Hohlfeld R, Kieseier BC. Immunobiology of muscle: advances in understanding an immunological microenvironment. Trends Immunol. 2005;26:373–80.

Wiggins OP, Barker JH, Martinez S, et al. On the ethics of face transplantation research. Am J Bioeth. 2004;4:1–12.

Wilhelmi BJ, Kang RH, Movassaghi K, Ganchi PA, et al. First successful replantation of face and scalp with single artery repair: model for face and scalp transplantation. Ann Plast Surg. 2003;50:535–40.

Wohlleben G, Hartung HP, Gold R. Humoral and cellular immune functions of cytokine-treated Schwann cells. Adv Exp Med Biol. 1999;468:151–6.

Worthington JE, Martin S, Al-Husaini DM, et al. Posttransplantation production of donor HLA-specific antibodies as a predictor of renal transplant outcome. Transplantation. 2003;75:1034–40.

Wyrick JD, Stern PJ. Secondary nerve reconstruction. Hand Clin. 1992;8:587–98.

Yazici I, Unal S, Siemionow M. Composite hemiface/calvaria transplantation model in rats. Plast Reconstr Surg. 2006;118:1321–7.

Yazici I, Carnevale K, Klimczak A, et al. A new rat model of maxilla allotransplantation. Ann Plast Surg. 2007;58:334–8.

Yi C, Guo S. Face transplantation: lessons so far. Lancet. 2009;374:177–8.

Yin JW, Matsuo JM, Hsieh CH, et al. Replantation of total avulsed scalp with microsurgery: experience of eight cases and literature review. J Trauma. 2008;64:796–802.

Zheng XX, Sanchez-Fueyo A, Domenig C, et al. The balance of deletion and regulation in allograft tolerance. Immunol Rev. 2003;196:75–84.

Zor F, Bozkurt M, Nair D, Siemionow M. A new composite midface allotransplantation model with sensory and motor reinnervation. Transpl Int. 2010;23:649–56.

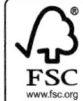